The GP Consultation Reimagined:

A Tale of Two Houses

For Clare, Ellen and Joe

The GP Consultation Reimagined:

A Tale of Two Houses

Martin Brunet

MA (Cantab), MBChB, MRCP, MRCGP, MSc

GP and GP Trainer, Binscombe Medical Centre, Godalming

Scion

Scion Publishing Limited

The Old Hayloft, Vantage Business Park, Bloxham Road, Banbury OX16 9UX, UK

www.scionpublishing.com

Important Note from the Publisher

The information contained within this book was obtained by Scion Publishing Ltd from sources believed by us to be reliable. However, while every effort has been made to ensure its accuracy, no responsibility for loss or injury whatsoever occasioned to any person acting or refraining from action as a result of information contained herein can be accepted by the authors or publishers.

Readers are reminded that medicine is a constantly evolving science and while the authors and publishers have ensured that all dosages, applications and practices are based on current indications, there may be specific practices which differ between communities. You should always follow the guidelines laid down by the manufacturers of specific products and the relevant authorities in the country in which you are practising.

Although every effort has been made to ensure that all owners of copyright material have been acknowledged in this publication, we would be pleased to acknowledge in subsequent reprints or editions any omissions brought to our attention.

Registered names, trademarks, etc. used in this book, even when not marked as such, are not to be considered unprotected by law.

Typeset by Medlar Publishing Solutions Pvt Ltd, India
Cover design by Andrew Magee Design Ltd
Printed in the UK by Ashford Colour Ltd

Last digit is the print number: 11

Contents

Foreword

If it's not careful, the general practice consultation could prove to be a frog. Not *any* old frog, you understand; I'm referring to the one in the story that, finding itself in a pan of water being heated from cold, fails to make the leap to safety that would have saved its life.

The tadpole that became a consultation-frog was spawned sometime in the 1950s, when British general practice, sick of being looked down on by toffee-nosed specialists, tried to pinpoint what it was that made generalism a specialty in its own right. An aphorism of Sir William Osler (ironically a hospital physician) caught the essence of it well, with only a tiny re-write: *'The good physician treats the disease; the great physician'* (or GP) *'treats the patient who has the disease'.*

Patient-centredness: an ungainly word and an easy slogan, but it means something that for 50 years has been at the heart of British general practice – the devotion of *all* one's skills, interpersonal as well as technical, to serving the interests of each individual patient. The consultation is where we put this aspiration into action. What we have come to regard as consulting skills – notwithstanding all the detail in which they have been written about, modelled and taught – are simply the way we communicate and enact our concern for the person sitting in the patient's chair.

Patient-centred consulting, then, is our frog in its saucepan. But the gas has been lit underneath it, and the poor creature is starting to feel the heat. The factors fuelling its predicament are a familiar litany. The chronic lack of capacity, resources and manpower in the NHS; the rising expectations of patients and the growing complexity of the problems they bring; doctors' understandable need for a more acceptable work/life balance, which inevitably limits continuity of care; a starry-eyed but misplaced faith in information technology and digital media as the means of salvation. Skilled consulting can cope with each of these trends individually, and indeed, can bring benefit to them. But cumulatively they can make nuanced, empathic, personalised care seem an outdated luxury, an impediment to what looks like progress. Watch out, frog; it'll soon be time to jump.

· · ·

Those three dots represent the passage of several days between my writing the foregoing and now picking up where I left off. In the interim,

Coronavirus has seized the nation by the throat. Amidst the fear and the danger and the tragedies are countless acts of heroism and kindness, and occasional ones of selfishness and folly. Although as I write it is far from clear what our institutions and way of life will look like in a post-pandemic world, one thing is certain – the virus has turned the heat up, and the consultation-frog is in serious trouble. Heat, as we know, speeds up reactions, and COVID-19 has hugely accelerated the trend towards depersonalisation of the consultation. Remote consulting, by phone or digital technology, has almost overnight become the new norm. Physical contact between GP and patient is severely curtailed, and emotional connection between them a fading memory. Phrases like 'Tell me all about it' die on the lips. All this is for the moment necessary, essential, life-saving. But at some point the outbreak will end; and what then?

The frog has jumped. But it lives. Post-COVID, things will never be the same again – except the things that will. One thing that won't have changed is human nature. And it is human nature, at times of pain, worry and distress, to seek the solace of – yes, of high-tech medicine; but also the solace of compassionate human understanding, as conveyed through the relationship with a GP who will have retained and nurtured the art of the consultation through dark times. People want to be not just cared *for*, but cared *about* …

… which is where Martin Brunet's book comes in. If we are to emerge from the current crisis with some kind of synergy between old and new ways of working, we need people who know how to look after scalded frogs. Martin is one such. He clearly loves consulting: its sweep, its depths, its intricacies, its incomparable rewards. His book will not teach you to improve your consultations. That is its great merit. Instead, it will encourage you to *learn* how to consult better. You do that by wanting to, by being inspired to follow your curiosity to the limit, and by being shown the abundance of satisfaction that awaits you if you do. The receding viral tsunami will create the opportunity for a rehumanising of our profession, a renaissance of the personal. Come that time, the commitment and thoughtfulness exemplified in this book will be crucial.

Roger Neighbour
OBE, MA, MB, BChir, DSc, FRCGP, FRCP, FRACGP

Bedmond, Hertfordshire
March 2020

Preface

It is nearly 30 years since I first ventured anxiously onto a hospital ward as a medical student, prepared to embark on that most terrifying of medical endeavours – talking to a real, live patient. My crisp new white coat and worried facial expression must have stood me apart from the actual doctors as I walked tentatively down the Nightingale ward on my mission; with every step I would secretly hope that my intended target would have visitors or be eating their lunch, so that I could scuttle away and live to fight another day.

A great deal has changed in those 30 years. For starters, I have found patients to be a whole lot less intimidating than I first feared, while white coats – with their wonderfully deep pockets and horrifyingly grubby sleeves – have long since had their day. There are new tests, such as the troponin T, and the ready availability of MRI scans, not to mention radically new treatments such as laparoscopic surgery and ground-breaking immunotherapy. One thing, however, has not changed one iota – the structure of how to clerk a patient is the same as it ever was. Some of the details behind the medical clerking model, and certainly the thinking behind it, may well have changed, but the basic structure – Presenting Complaint; History of Presenting Complaint; Past Medical and Surgical History, etc. – has not varied. It was how my seniors were taught, how they taught me and how medical students are taught today.

There are two good reasons for this remarkable consistency over so many decades. The first is that, by and large, the model for taking a medical history in the hospital setting is fit for purpose – it achieves its intended aim, which is to gather a complete analysis of a problem and ensure there are no gaps. The second is that it has such an identifiable and repeatable structure that it is easy to see if someone is *doing it right* – which means it is easy to teach and easy to test; anyone who decides to take a history in a different way would be doing it wrong, marked down in examinations and corrected until they got it right. This makes the medical clerking model, for better or worse, both resistant to erosion and incapable of evolution.

Not so in general practice; the GP consultation is an altogether more slippery beast. There is no *right* way to do it, making it hard to teach and even harder to define in an examination; at first glance it can seem to lack any structure at all. Ask a medical student how they take a medical history and they will rattle through the structure they follow in an instant, giving the same answer as the next student. Ask a GP the same question and they will almost certainly hesitate, if they can answer it at all, and the answers from a group of GPs will be as varied as their political viewpoints. Many will quote consultation models that have influenced them – such as Neighbour[1], Balint[2] or Pendleton[3], but these giants in the history of the GP consultation will be exactly that – influencers, just as an artist might be influenced by learning from the Grand Masters – with ideas learnt, techniques borrowed, and methods adapted for their own use. Few GPs would ever say that they follow any one consultation model in its entirety, and none would do so in a rigid manner for every consultation. In fact, many of the consultation 'models' that have been described – such as Balint, and Byrne and Long[4], for instance – were not so much a structure that GPs should follow as an analysis of what GPs were actually doing, in an attempt to understand it. What makes the GP consultation so dynamic, so exciting and so altogether bewildering, therefore, is that it has formed through a process of evolution over the last 70 years, and stubbornly resisted attempts to pin it down or put it neatly into a box.

This book has been born out of my own attempts to wrestle with the complexities and frustrations of trying to communicate with my own patients, and the challenge of teaching the GP consultation to trainees in my practice and over nearly ten years in my role as Programme Director on the Guildford GP Training scheme. As a formulation of my own thoughts and ideas, it is not an academic work; nor is it evidence-based, nor an account of the rich heritage we already have on this topic (for which there are excellent works already published – such as Tim Usherwood's eloquent *Understanding the Consultation*[5] and Liz Moulton's superb, accessible and up-to-date *The Naked Consultation*[6]).

Attempting to write about the consultation at all is an inescapably humbling undertaking, since your own failings and inadequacies come to the front of your mind when you consider how you would like to consult compared to the realities of day-to-day life in general practice. We all have

1. Neighbour, R. (2015) *The Inner Consultation*, 2nd edition. CRC Press.

2. Balint, M. (1957) *The Doctor, his Patient and the Illness*. Pitman Medical.

3. Pendleton, D., Schofield, T., Tate, P. and Havelock, P. (1984) *The Consultation: an approach to learning and teaching*. Oxford University Press.

4. Byrne, P. and Long, B. (1976) *Doctors Talking to Patients*. Her Majesty's Stationery Office.

5. Usherwood, T. (1999) *Understanding the Consultation: evidence, theory, and practice*. Open University Press.

6. Moulton, L. (2016) *The Naked Consultation: a practical guide to primary care consultation skills*, 2nd edition. CRC Press.

times when we are tired, distracted, frustrated, irritated, overworked and, at the end of a busy duty day, downright frazzled. However, we all also have consultations where we get it right, where we know that the patient has left feeling listened to, understood and fully satisfied with the outcome and – at least until we call in the next patient – we can remind ourselves that this is why we come to work. We won't get it right all the time, but since truly effective consulting is what can, should and does happen in general practice, taking the time to consider what such consultations look like seems well worth the effort.

What I hope this book will prove to be is a new and creative way of thinking about the consultation that is suitable for the 21st century – where patients rightly expect to be centrally involved in their own care, but also want to work in partnership with their doctor and not be left to make all the decisions on their own. I have hesitated to call *Two Houses* a model for the consultation, although that is one way of thinking of it and you will find me using that term. It may be better to think of it as an *imagining* of the consultation, one that may help us to reconsider what is happening between doctor and patient, and so to use this understanding to shape the dynamic and improve both communication and decision-making. In order to be of the greatest value, *Two Houses* cannot be a model to reach for once in a while but needs to have something to say for every consultation, whether the problem is very straightforward and simple, or complex, seemingly insoluble and ongoing. Equally, it has to remain relevant to 21st-century settings for the consultation, since we are now as likely to communicate with our patients on the telephone, via email or even via an app as in a traditional face-to-face appointment. I have kept these goals in mind as the model has shaped over the last few years, but it will be for the reader to judge how well I have achieved such ambitions aims.

I hope *The GP Consultation Reimagined: a tale of two houses* will be of interest to established GPs, as well as GP trainees and GP educators, and also to the increasing numbers of nurses, paramedics, physicians' associates and pharmacists who are equally engaged in this business of consulting as they help to shape the modern world of general practice.

Acknowledgements

I am particularly grateful to be part of a vibrant and supportive group of GP Trainers on the Guildford scheme. This fabulous group of doctors has been through some highs and lows over the years, but we have always been there for each other as we have laughed and cried together. For me personally, it was the enthusiasm and encouragement of these colleagues that gave me the courage to step out and start writing, and I am very grateful to them all. I would particularly like to thank Hamish Whitaker for asking me to teach on the consultation to established GPs, the catalytic event that crystallised my thinking about the consultation and made me realise that, without planning to, I had come up with a new consultation model.

The Guildford scheme would have been much poorer without the unique contribution of each of the fellow Programme Directors that I was lucky enough to work with over my 10 years there, and so I would like to thank Simon Dunbar, Cath Humphrys, Leslie Campbell, Fiona Groom and Debra Harper for being such stimulating and inspiring company as we taught together. Thanks to Fiona and Debra in particular for the grace with which they handled the news that I was to step down and abandon them! Thanks also to Donna Stevens for being the glue that held everything together.

I am very fortunate to work with a wonderful team at Binscombe and am deeply grateful to my fellow partners, past and present, and also the other doctors, nurses, reception and admin team that make Binscombe such a special and happy place to work. I have also been fortunate enough to work with an exciting range of trainees over the years, each and every one of whom has taught me far more than they know or realise.

I am very grateful to Jonathan Ray at Scion for believing in *Two Houses* from the outset and for being so responsive to my endless questions, as well as to Clare Boomer for keeping me posted at every stage as she took me through the fascinating process that is publication. I am grateful to Roger Neighbour for standing up for the consultation at every turn, and deeply humbled that he agreed to write the Foreword for this book.

Fundamental to who I am is my family, so my biggest thanks go to Clare, Ellen and Joe for their love and encouragement and for being the best. Also to Clare, Ellen and my sister Carol for being such astute proofreaders— women who really know their 'practice' from their 'practise'!

About the author

Martin Brunet is a GP and GP Trainer at Binscombe Medical Centre in Godalming. He was a Programme Director on the Guildford GP training scheme from 2009 to 2019 when he stepped down from the role in order to write this book. He has blogged extensively in the past on his own practice website as well as for *Pulse* magazine, with a particular interest in overdiagnosis and overmedicalisation, but his primary passion has always been for effective communication in the consultation. He will be running teaching courses on the *Two Houses Model*, and details of these courses, as well as links to all the *Two Houses Guides*, can be found on his website, www.twohousesgp.com. He enjoys a good chat on Twitter @docmartin68.

Chapter 1

The GP consultation in the ICE age

A personal journey in the consultation

My own experience of communicating with patients was firmly rooted in the hospital model. Apart from a rather disorientating five-week placement in general practice as a final-year medical student, I learnt everything in a hospital setting, following my house officer year by pursuing a path into general medicine, including two years as that most pitied of hospital creatures, the medical registrar. I enjoyed my interactions with patients, and it was the loss of this front-line contact as I became more senior that led to me 'seeing the light' and heading into general practice. Before making this transition I liked to think that I was a reasonably empathetic hospital doctor who valued good communication, but when I started GP training the idea that I should actively ask patients what they thought, or what they wanted, was nothing short of a revelation to me.

Even now I cringe as I remember a patient whom I saw over a number of months in a medical clinic. He suffered from debilitating headaches, and, while I remember nothing at all of the clinical scenario, I can still see the frustration on his face as, time and again, he came back to tell me that my previous great idea for treating his headaches had proven no better than the last one, and he was still in pain. At no point did it occur to me to ask him what he thought, what he was hoping we might do next, or to consider that his headaches might be anything other than a clearly defined clinical condition. No one had taught me to think differently, and I completely lacked the skills to navigate medically

At no point did it occur to me to ask my patient what *he* thought

unexplained symptoms. Learning for the first time how to enquire about someone's ideas, concerns and expectations (ICE), hearing about the difference between illness and disease, and learning that taking an holistic approach could help me to understand the unique experience of illness my patient was living through, was like having scales fall from my eyes.

It was exciting, frustrating and bewildering as I started to see medicine differently and learnt to adapt to this new way of interacting with patients. Part of me was angry that I had never been taught this before, while I was also disappointed in myself for not working more of it out on my own, but mostly I lapped it up, and tried hard to adapt to this new way of thinking.

I loved learning about consultation models – I was mercifully free from the pressure to learn them for an examination. This is not the case for current GP trainees who have to study the models in the abstract for their Applied Knowledge Test as part of the Membership of the Royal College of General Practitioners (MRCGP) examination, something I believe has destroyed much of the interest trainees might have had in their heritage. We stand on the shoulders of giants, but the requirement to name these giants in a multiple choice exam has, regrettably, reduced their wisdom to mundane facts to be learnt today and quickly forgotten. The time to learn about the consultation is not with a textbook and a set of past papers, but in the hot seat with the patient, where, inspired by what you have learnt in theory, you see what actually works in practice. I remember one consultation ending with my patient standing up, saying to me, *"And am I happy? No!"* and walking out before I had a chance to answer – there was a lot of learning from that one! Like all trainees before me and after, I have had the predictable retort to my clumsy attempt to find out their ideas about their illness, *"Well, I don't know, aren't you meant to be the doctor?"*. And yet I had unmistakable triumphs along the way that only occurred because I had tried something new, such as patients who told me that they were worried about something which was so left field and medically bizarre that I would never would have thought of it, or so embarrassing that they never would have mentioned it without being given space to express their fears.

However, I struggled to remember the consultation models. The hospital model was easy – there was only one model, it had a clear structure and every time you wrote up your notes you recorded each of the headings so that mere repetition drummed them home; and I had spent the last nine years doing it time and again. Now there were more consultation models than I could count, and the headings were often nebulous, like 'Establishes Rapport' – how exactly do I know when I am doing that? How do I know when it is done and I can move on to the next bit? I could remember parts of several models – ICE from Pendleton[1] and Safety-netting from Neighbour[2] stood out in particular – but I could not remember the rest. Was that because they weren't important, or were they just too obvious to remember, or was I

---

1. Pendleton, D., Schofield, T., Tate, P. and Havelock, P. (1984) *The Consultation: an approach to learning and teaching.* Oxford University Press.

2. Neighbour, R. (2015) *The Inner Consultation*, 2nd edition. CRC Press.

just not good at them? I could remember aspects of some others, like 'Flash Points' and 'The Doctor as Drug' from Balint[3], but these didn't seem like a model you could follow at all, more an observation of some of the apparently random things that might – or might not – happen in a consultation.

I gravitated towards Neighbour, partly because I enjoyed his writing, but also, I am sure, because he only had five points for me to remember – Connecting, Summarising, Handing Over, Safety-netting and House-keeping, and the last one of those didn't even happen during the consultation, so that left just four to worry about. I loved (and still do) his interest in the very first part of the consultation, that part of Connecting that he called the Opening Gambit and the Curtain-raiser. What was magical about these two concepts was that I didn't have to do anything other than observe them; they didn't involve a question or an action I had to take and were entirely the patient's responsibility. The Opening Gambit is the well-rehearsed opening line the patient has planned to say – like *"It's my back again, doctor"* or *"I think I'm cracking up"*, while the Curtain-raiser is the random comment that might pop out more spontaneously – such as *"I usually see Dr Patel"* or *"You're running late"*. I found the patient frequently gave me useful information in these one-liners, if I learned to notice it, and loved the fact that I didn't have to worry about whether or not this would happen – the patient would say these things whether I wanted them to or not.

> **What was magical about the Opening Gambit and the Curtain-raiser was that I didn't have to do anything other than observe them**

Much as I felt inspired by Neighbour, however, I struggled to 'follow' his model. I usually had a stab at safety-netting, but would frequently forget to summarise, or I would think about summarising, but it just wouldn't seem appropriate – do you really need to summarise when all you've done is check a mole that is entirely benign, or done a pill check with someone who is completely happy with their contraception? And how did I incorporate ICE, when it seemed important, but wasn't overtly part of Neighbour's model?

Consulting in the ICE age

And so we come to ICE. Since Pendleton and colleagues first raised the idea that doctors should endeavour to find out the ideas, concerns and expectations of the patient in 1984, this concept has probably influenced the practice of the consultation more than any other; usually for the better,

---

3. Balint, M. (1957) *The Doctor, his Patient and the Illness*. Pitman Medical.

but sometimes for the worse. That's why the title of this first chapter is *The GP consultation in the ICE age*, because it has become part of the established order and, like most good ideas, it has been both used and abused over the years. Most medical students have heard of ICE, even if they have never heard of Pendleton, and most GP trainees recognise its importance. As a concept, it has a great deal of merit – it has to be a fundamentally good objective to find out what the patient is thinking. If the patient has an *idea* of what the problem is, the doctor can best work with or challenge this idea if they know what the patient is thinking; where the patient is worried about what is going on with their body, the doctor can only relieve their *concern* – or share that they are concerned too – if they know what it is; and if a patient has a clear idea of what they *expect* to happen next and the doctor shows no signs of doing it, then that can lead to a very dysfunctional consultation indeed.

I am a great believer in ICE, but have also encountered many frustrations with it. The Clinical Skills Assessment (CSA) of the MRCGP has to shoulder some of the blame here. For those unfamiliar with the delights of the CSA, this exam is probably the single most stressful experience of a GP trainee's whole career. The trainee is required to see thirteen simulated patients in a row, with each 'patient' being an actor playing out a particular scenario, and each consultation being closely observed and marked by an unsmiling examiner, complete with clipboard and pen. While it is certainly important to assess a trainee's clinical skills, and the CSA is not the worst way of doing this, it is a major factor in why trainees take less interest in the historical consultation models than they used to – because ultimately the model they all want to perfect is not a consultation model at all, but the how-to-get-through-the-CSA model. It is a shame, since simply learning good general consultation skills will get any decent trainee comfortably through the exam, but it is understandable nevertheless and a powerful, if depressing, example of how assessment can drive learning. While there is not a tick box on any CSA marking sheet for 'has done ICE', the exam does expect the trainees to demonstrate that they have managed to elicit the patient's health beliefs in some way, and this has sometimes led to the practice of 'ICE for ICE's sake'. If ICE becomes an objective in itself, it can easily become formulaic and stilted, or the trainee uncovers useful information, but then fails to do anything with it – it is like listening with a stethoscope and ignoring your findings, or asking someone what they want for their birthday and then getting them something completely different.

Rosamund Snow, the *BMJ* Patient editor, eloquently describes what it is like to "be ICE'd" in this way in a short but powerful essay in the *BMJ*[4].

---

4. Snow, R. (2016) I never asked to be ICE'd. *BMJ*, **354**: 1–2.

She understands why doctors might want to find out this information, but wonders whether anyone has ever asked patients how such questions sound, or might make them feel. She describes how being asked what you think is wrong with you can either feel like the doctor has no idea themselves, or that they know exactly what is going on and are testing you in some complex game where only they know the rules. Her short paper is unsettling, and an important read for anyone trying to grasp the noble principles behind ICE, without handling it so clumsily that the patient gets stung.

Far more common than seeing ICE done badly, however, is not seeing it done at all. Again and again I have seen excellent trainees simply not make any attempt to find out what the patient is thinking. My frustrated response to this has been to work harder at teaching ICE, but perhaps it is better to try to understand why our trainees find it so difficult in the first place. My suspicion is that if I were to watch my own practice, I would also be disappointed by how well I use ICE; perhaps it is not just a lack of effective teaching that underpins this. Are doctors (myself included) just not interested in what their patients are thinking, or are there other reasons why an effective attempt at ICE is not the norm? I think there are several reasons for this, and the first is simply the overwhelming challenge that general practice poses, especially at the start of training. The breadth of clinical knowledge required, the pressure to come up with any plan at all – especially as a single clinician rather than when operating as part of a wider clinical team in a hospital setting – can be so great that the trainee is just relieved when they themselves have an idea of what might be happening and can think of a plan to deal with it. Is it any wonder that finding out the patient's health beliefs might get squeezed out in the process?

One big failing with asking ICE-related questions is that the returns are not that great

Once the trainee gains in confidence, these stresses will recede; they often develop excellent skills at patient-centred medicine, and will sometimes use ICE, but not always – why is this? Pressures of time probably play a large factor, but one big failing with ICE is that, frankly, when asking a direct ICE-related question, the returns are not that great – by which I mean that most patients don't have a neatly defined idea, concern or expectation, and very few indeed have a clear idea on all three.

It doesn't take much skill to refine your question and avoid the impression that you have no ideas yourself; for example:

> *"Before I make any suggestions, did you have any thoughts about what we might do next?"*

> *"I'm always interested in what you are thinking, did you have any thoughts about where we might go with this?"*

The problem is that, although questions like these do work reasonably well, even then people will often answer with, *"No, not really"*. They may have an expectation of *something*, but they are not sure what; or they might be worried that if they make a suggestion then that is what they will get, whether or not it is the best option and they don't want to colour the doctor's views; or maybe they don't want to appear stupid with a daft idea, or seem like a worrier and give the doctor the wrong impression. And it matters if a question has a low return rate – because the doctor learns to stop asking it. There seems a world of difference between ICE that comes out naturally in the back and forth of a responsive conversation between doctor and patient, based on active listening and close attention to cues and non-verbal hints, and a more forced, unsolicited enquiry.

Finally, many of our consultations just don't seem to 'require' ICE; very simple conditions and routine check-ups may not warrant an in-depth enquiry into health beliefs, so we learn to ask about ICE only in the more complex cases, or where we suspect there is a hidden agenda – but then get out of the habit of doing it, so may forget about it when it would be more useful. This is even more true when it comes to follow-up appointments and routine reviews – how does ICE work when someone comes for their blood pressure check-up? It may

There is much more to patient-centred consulting than simply eliciting ICE

have a role, clearly, but it is not as straightforward as when a patient attends with a classic presenting problem. Indeed, talking to a trainee recently, she said how different it was consulting having got the CSA exam out of the way. The 'CSA model', she explained, only really applies when a patient first presents with a new problem, and so much of what she was now doing was much more 'real' than that: such as appointments spent mostly listening to what it is like to live with long-standing, seemingly insoluble problems; chronic disease management; or journeying with someone through a period of depression, bereavement or a protracted illness. She is absolutely right; the artificial emphasis on consultations that 'fit' the CSA does little to prepare the trainee for so much else that can occur in the GP consultation, and threatens to strip the joy of consulting in the process.

Part of what I hope to cover in this book addresses my concern that ICE, while very worthy, is too narrow a definition of what a patient may be thinking, and of what really matters – there is much more to patient-centred consulting than simply eliciting ICE. So, while trying to do ICE well will always be a skill worth developing, I think we need something simpler, something easier to grasp and more applicable to any and every consultation, and something that won't be so dependent on the health literacy of the patient – it's a tall order!

Chapter 2

Two Houses – a new model for the consultation

Thrown into the mix

"Do you think I should have a flu jab?"

"A flu jab?"

"Yes, I just wondered if it would be wise…"

"Are you in one of the at-risk groups?"

"No… I don't think so."

As a consultation, the above exchange is hardly riveting stuff. There is no need to formulate a diagnosis, no symptomatology to explore, no examination to undertake. As a vignette in general practice, however, it is typical of the sort of question that is thrown into the mix of what we see every day – probably not as the only reason for attendance (wouldn't that be easy?!) but brought up by the patient in a while-I'm-here sort of way. Despite its lack of drama, it is worth considering how we might respond to such a question.

One entirely appropriate response would be to consider the guidance on vaccinations from the Department of Health and, having established that this young man is indeed not in any of the at-risk groups, to inform him that his risk is low and so it is not worth him having the jab. The problem with guidelines, however, is that they are always incomplete, since they cannot include the individual context of the patient we have in front of us – they are like a jigsaw puzzle with several of the most crucial pieces missing.

In this scenario, the doctor might try to find these missing pieces by asking a question like, *"Why do you ask?"*

If we hypothesise as to why a healthy young man might want to consider a flu jab it is not difficult to envisage several scenarios. Perhaps he just doesn't like the idea of flu and would like to avoid it? Maybe he is more worried about flu than he needs to be – a friend of his could have ended up in hospital, but if that friend had type 1 diabetes perhaps that was why he got so ill. It could be that there is someone else to be worried about – has this man just become a dad and knows his partner had the flu jab while she was pregnant, so should he also try to protect their baby? Or perhaps he lives with his parents and his mum is just about to start chemotherapy, so he doesn't want to bring flu into the family home. On the other hand, it could be that his risk is low, but he can't afford to get ill this winter: he's getting married / going trekking / about to have his big breakthrough in the world of athletics / due to have a long-awaited operation. The possibilities are endless, and the importance of such events is entirely for him to know and, if we are to answer his question in a way that is helpful, for us to find out.

Twitter is a great way to snoop in on other people's conversations, and one such conversation I overheard is worth sharing here. A consultant surgeon asked the Twittersphere to explain shared decision-making to him, and the best response I saw was from a GP in Wales called Sally Lewis – a compassionate and level-headed GP who often has wise things to say. She described shared decision-making as "asking the person what matters to them and then figuring out together the best way to achieve (it)". Putting aside any concerns that a consultant had to ask this question in the first place – shared decision-making should never be seen as solely in the domain of primary care – Sally's answer is the key to answering this young man's question. If we can find out what matters to him, we might be able to help him evaluate the merits or otherwise of a flu jab, be it possible on the NHS or something he would have to pay for. What is more, it strikes me that Sally's response went beyond the original question on shared decision-making and contains something of the essence of general practice.

Many of the established consultation models contain the idea that we have to find some things out, and then do something about it – some examples of this are included in the table below:

Model	Finding things out	Doing something about it
Byrne and Long[1]	• Discovering the reason for attendance • Verbal and/or physical examination	• Doctor and/or patient consider the condition • Detail further treatment or investigation
Pendleton[2]	Understanding the problem • Nature and history of the problem • Aetiology • Ideas, concerns and expectations • Effects of the problem	• Choose an appropriate action for each problem • Share decisions and responsibility
Neighbour[3]	• Connecting • Summarising	• Handing over
Calgary–Cambridge[4]	• Initiating the session • Gathering information • Building the relationship	• Explanation and planning

The *Two Houses* model

Finding things out and deciding what to do are clearly important in historical consultation models. The *Two Houses* model is a new model of the consultation that places these ideas centre stage as the fundamental essence of every consultation. Crucial to the model is that these should not be considered as *tasks* for the doctor to complete at a given point in time, but as *objectives* to be achieved throughout the consultation, with doctor and patient constantly working together towards these twin goals.

1. Byrne, P. and Long, B. (1976) *Doctors Talking to Patients: a study of the verbal behaviour of general practitioners consulting in their surgeries.* Her Majesty's Stationery Office.

2. Pendleton, D., Schofield, T., Tate, P. and Havelock, P. (2003) *The New Consultation: developing doctor–patient communication.* Oxford University Press.

3. Neighbour, R. (2015) *The Inner Consultation,* 2nd edition. CRC Press.

4. Silverman, J., Kurtz, S. and Draper, J. (2013) *Skills for Communicating with Patients,* 3rd edition. CRC Press.

Work out what matters

I prefer the term 'work out what matters' to 'find out what matters' or to 'ask the person what matters to them' contained in Sally's tweet, since the doctor needs to be very active in working out what matters; it is hard work! For example, what matters to the patient might be to know if their heart is OK in light of the chest pains they have been getting – but they do not have the knowledge to know how concerned they should be about their symptoms. The doctor, therefore, needs to take a careful history to work out if there is a heart problem or not. On the other hand, the patient might say that what matters to them is to have some painkillers for their chest pain, but the doctor learns that what really matters is that the pain is more serious than this and could well be angina. In other words, working out what matters is not just a matter of asking the patient, but combining this with doing some serious 'doctoring'. Patient-centred medicine is never a matter of just 'doing what the patient wants', but involves the application of medical knowledge, leadership and responsibility by the doctor, while always being focused on the unique individual we are working with.

> **Working out what matters is not just a matter of asking the patient, but combining this with doing some serious 'doctoring'**

Decide together what to do about it

The crucial word here is 'together'; many a well-worked management plan flounders when doctor and patient are no longer on the same page when it comes to decision-making. The doctor may become frustrated when the patient rejects their entirely reasonable treatment, while the patient may be annoyed that their own thoughts have gone unheard or been dismissed. When there is agreement between doctor and patient, however, and a shared understanding has been achieved (see *Chapter 9* for more on the importance of a shared understanding) then the consultation can reach a very satisfactory conclusion.

The Two Houses

Distilling the consultation down to the bare bones of these two objectives has the great advantage of simplicity; there is some hope that I will be able to keep in mind a model when there are only two things to consider! Instead of remembering to complete certain tasks in the consultation, I can simply keep asking myself: 'What is it that matters here?' and 'Are we working together on what to do next?'. The skills required to effectively achieve these objectives, however, are much more complex. For instance, while we may aspire to be patient-centred as we work out what matters, we may find that we constantly default to ignoring the patient's perspective, or our desire to work with the patient in formulating a plan may not be borne out in practice if we lack the skills to achieve a shared understanding.

In the *Two Houses* model we shall consider the two key objectives of the consultation as two imaginary houses, to be explored with the patient:

> The *House of Discovery* is where we work out what matters.

> The *House of Decision* is where we decide together what to do about it.

The consultation usually takes each house in turn, progressing from *Discovery* to *Decision*, with a similar amount of time spent in each. Central to this idea is that both houses belong to the patient; the model is so embedded in the patient's life and story that it is inherently patient-centred. The patient is not invited to bring their contribution into the doctor's domain, but the doctor chooses to respond to the patient's request to enter their unique houses of *Discovery* and *Decision*, and to work with them on their terms and in their territory.

> **Both houses belong to the patient; the model is so embedded in the patient's life and story that it is inherently patient-centred**

The *House of Discovery*

The *House of Discovery* (see the inside front cover) is the patient's story; it contains the full narrative of their life, their family and social context, hopes, dreams and fears, as well as the story of why they have attended at that time and in that place – the specific symptoms they present with as well as the physical signs the doctor might elicit. This house is entirely familiar to the patient, since it is the life they have lived and are living, but in the same way that my kitchen appliances are all familiar to me even though I only have a partial idea of their technical operating specifications, so the patient's familiarity with their own narrative does not always equate to a full understanding of what their story – and their symptoms in particular – actually means. Initially, while doctors can have a great deal of expertise in the general workings of a patient's house, the particular house of each individual patient is largely unknown to the doctor. The patient's notes may help to give a rough framework to the life in front of us, but this is the briefest of sketches and we need to start listening to their story as they permit us entry to their house and start to show us around. Over time, the doctor can build upon what they have learned and develop a shared understanding of the patient's context, so that they are not always starting from scratch. This is one aspect of general practice that can be bewildering to new trainees when they sit in with an established GP; observing the knowledge the doctor has built up of the patient's life, illnesses and relationships can seem like starting a box-set drama in the middle of series four with no explanation of what has gone before, making the structure of the consultation hard for the trainee to follow. This continuity and prior knowledge, however, is one of the great strengths of primary care; it makes the *House of Discovery* easier to navigate, but the doctor never knows how much more there is to explore. There may be multiple hallways which are as yet uncharted, or even entire suites of rooms the patient has not thought to take the doctor into, or to where they have, so far, denied access.

> Observing a GP consultation can seem like starting a box-set drama in the middle of series 4 without having seen series 1–3

The *House of Decision*

The *House of Decision*, on the other hand (see the inside back cover), while it still belongs to the patient, is usually much less familiar to them. Instead of exploring areas of the house in order to discover the patient's story, doctor and patient find their way around this house on the basis of the decisions they may choose to make. Its rooms are full of medical knowledge, explanations and guidelines; there are complex, technical rooms to navigate, rooms containing treatment options as simple as an emollient cream or as serious as open-heart surgery, rooms that can be ignored and rooms that have to be faced. It is the doctor's job to have a sure knowledge of this house – or at least to know where to find the plans for the areas they are less familiar with – and their role is to help the patient navigate it successfully, operating like a skilled and flexible tour guide. Just as the doctor gradually becomes familiar with the *House of Discovery*, so the patient's journey leads to them learning to find their way around the *House of Decision*. Some patients have a head start here, since any prior medical knowledge will help them to have an understanding of its layout. Even without any medical background, however, the patient will gradually become familiar with some areas of this house – they will have tried that medication before, they know how well that steroid injection worked in the past, and so on. The reason for this is that wherever we end up in the *House of Decision* will become incorporated into the patient's narrative – and so will be part of the *House of Discovery* the next time we or another health professional see them. This interaction between the two houses has a huge impact on how the patient approaches the second house – some will be keen to dive headlong into action and medical intervention, and may need help to protect them from the dangers of overdiagnosis and overtreatment, while others will have large areas of this house that they consider to be 'no-go' areas; maybe they shy away from blood tests due to a needle phobia, or are terrified of hospitals, sceptical of the orthodox medical model or reluctant to consider medication as they are not a 'pill popper'.

This interaction works both ways, since the patient's story will not only affect how they feel about the rooms in the second house but will often determine what is within its walls in the first place. The doctor might believe, for instance, that the patient's health would improve if they could get more exercise, but how can the doctor know what form this might take? For my own part, for instance, I could easily be persuaded to do more walking or gardening but going to a gym to work out has never appealed to me; it is only by taking time in my own *House of Discovery* that a doctor could know this and help me find my way to the room marked 'gardening', ignoring the 'gym' room next to it, since I have no interest in venturing in there. Or a doctor might help their patient to recognise that they are overly stressed, but what will help them to destress? Making changes at work? Taking time to exercise? Finding a creative hobby? The alternatives are endless, and as unique as the patient before them. This is just one reason why it is important to resist the notion that the *House of Decision* is the doctor's domain. The temptation to get to this part of the consultation and simply lead the patient to the 'right' room, and so the 'right' decision, can be very great, but the best solutions are often the ones that the patient finds for themself, or certainly where the patient has played a central role in their formation.

> **It is important to resist the notion that the *House of Decision* is the doctor's domain**

Navigating these two houses is a complex business and requires a wide range of skills. Just as a surveyor would bring technical equipment with them when going to survey a house, or a surgeon would have a range of scalpels, forceps and swabs laid out on the sterile tray next to them before they operate, so a GP needs to be equipped with the tools of their trade. The next chapter will consider what goes into this GP toolbox, while much of the rest of the book will be concerned with the detail within the two houses.

Chapter 3

The GP toolbox

In her critique on "being ICE'd"[1], as discussed in *Chapter 1*, Rosamund Snow contrasts the unpleasant experience of having her ideas, concerns and expectations explored in a clumsy manner, with a different encounter where she felt the doctor had "gold standard communication skills". Snow reports how well she felt listened to and how the doctor's primary focus was answering the questions Snow had asked. She also remarks on how well this doctor shared her thoughts as she went along so that they could discuss them together, an approach that made Snow feel more able to share her own thoughts and worries. What is especially noteworthy about Snow's commentary on this interaction is that she felt that she had started to trust this doctor in the first fifteen seconds. ***Fifteen seconds?!***

What was the doctor doing so well in those first moments that trust was apparent at such an early stage? Snow doesn't tell us, unfortunately, but it is a worthwhile reminder of how much we communicate with every word and action, and therefore how it is worth fully engaging in this process if we want to reach a good outcome for the patient.

Communication is one of the most fundamental aspects of being human and, if we are to truly master this art, we can learn a great deal by becoming keen observers of people, noting how they interact and learning from it, storing away things that work and spotting the traps and pitfalls that we might fall into. We should conduct such observations when we are out in the world, waiting at a bus stop or eating in a restaurant, but we can also learn from some of the true masters in the art of communication (see *Box 3.1*).

---

1. Snow, R. (2016) I never asked to be ICE'd. *BMJ*, **354:** 1–2.

Box 3.1 Expert communicating

The talk show host Michael Parkinson is a real expert in communication – after 25 years of interviewing celebrities on his show we can conclude that he has probably learnt a thing or two! A good example of some of the skills he uses is an interview he conducted with Steve Coogan, who plays the fictional character Alan Partridge. Here is a transcript of how the interview begins:

Michael Parkinson:	*"Welcome"*
Steve Coogan:	*"Thank you"*
Michael Parkinson:	*"Bring us up to date on Mr Partridge"*
Steve Coogan:	*"Well he's no longer living in a Travel Tavern... he's now living in a static home..."*
Michael Parkinson:	**(sitting forward, nods)**
Steve Coogan:	*"... not... not a caravan..."*
Michael Parkinson:	*"No"*
Steve Coogan:	*"... a static home"*
Michael Parkinson:	*"A static home"*
Steve Coogan:	*"There's a difference. Next to his house that's being built."*
Michael Parkinson:	*"And his job?"*

What is interesting is to see how little Parkinson actually says, and yet it is clear that he is in complete control of the interview. The simple word 'no' highlights to both Coogan and the audience that he has clocked the importance that the new living arrangements are not to be confused with a caravan, while his echoing of Coogan's description of a static home imprints this image in the mind of the viewer. When Parkinson wants to move the conversation on, he asks about Partridge's job with supreme efficiency with the simple question, *"And his job?"*

While written prose usually has to be grammatically correct, and our children are taught how to construct a full sentence, real-life dialogue rarely sticks to the rules. By staying so succinct, Parkinson is able to direct the conversation without taking over or getting in the way of Coogan being the one on centre stage. He can ask a question with three simple words and not a verb in sight, but the meaning is clear and the flow of the interview is maintained. While our context is very different, these are all skills for the GP to learn.

The golden minute

So, if we are to have any hope of building trust within fifteen seconds, what is a GP to do in the opening salvo of a consultation? The influential study by Beckman and Frankel[2] reminds us not to interrupt the patient, with the headline statistic that physicians allowed their patients an average of only 18 seconds before doing just that. What, however, do we mean by interrupting? We are told that we should respect the 'golden minute' at the beginning of the consultation and give the patient time to speak, but what do we doctors do during that time? Respecting this 'patient time' does not mean that we simply sit passively without any form of communication. Like Michael Parkinson, we need to engage in communication from the outset, with a nod of the head here, an affirming *"right"* or *"OK"* there; and body language that supports the patient in their attempt to communicate with us. Before we ask a question in these first moments of the consultation, we should think carefully about how it might affect the patient's flow and use such questions like a gentle hand on the tiller, resisting any attempt to completely change direction.

Take a tip from Michael Parkinson and think carefully before you rush in with a question!

"That's OK"

Adam had sat in the waiting room for a while rehearsing what to say, but he just got more wound up the more he tried to think about it; it had been years since he'd been in the doctor's surgery and even booking in had seemed an ordeal. In the end, when the doctor called him in, he just blurted out *"I don't know how to start."*

"That's OK," came the reply.

Not raised eyebrows or a sigh at another patient who didn't know how to do this, or even a non-committal *"OK"*, but *"That's OK"*; it was OK that he didn't know where to start; she was OK with that. And so it all came out: the stress at work, the chest pain that he knew really wasn't his heart – but hadn't his colleague just had a heart attack? – and that was part of why work was so stressful; and the new baby; and poor sleep; and money worries; and he knew he was drinking more than he should. It wasn't very ordered, but it all came out and she listened. He couldn't tell how he knew she listened, but he just knew, and when he'd finished she said *"I'm glad you've come."*

Adam paused for a moment. He still didn't know what to do next, or where this would lead to, but he knew he was glad he'd come too.

2. Beckman, H. B. and Frankel, R. M. (1984) The effect of physician behaviour on the collection of data. *Annals of Internal Medicine*, **101:** 692–696.

Dialogue in the consultation

One way of seeing dialogue in the consultation is to envisage it like the passing of a baton between the patient and the doctor:

- first the patient speaks, and is allowed to speak without interruption
- then they pass the baton to the doctor, who takes the lead for a while before passing it back to the patient.

Indeed, Larsen and Neighbour[3] recommend considering the consultation in three parts:

- The Patient's Part
- The Doctor's Part
- The Shared Part.

There are benefits in thinking this way, since this is a natural pattern for the consultation and it can remind the doctor to give the patient time at the beginning and ensure they are brought back in at the end. Larsen and Neighbour are certainly not advocating that the doctor and patient must remain passive in each other's 'part', but there is a danger that this slightly artificial division of the consultation could reduce the sense of a shared journey running seamlessly through the entire encounter.

An alternative analogy is to consider the consultation more like a dance, and, oddly enough, like a dance on the television show *Strictly Come Dancing*. If the show has never been part of your Saturday evenings then bear with me, and be reassured that there will be no need to understand the visual imagery of the *paso doble,* the importance of a well-executed *fleckerl,* or how to tell a *salsa* from a *samba*. What is fundamental to the show is that each dancing couple consists of a professional dancer and a celebrity; the celebrity may be a complete novice to the whole concept of moving their body to music, or they may have a background in the performing arts or and even in dance itself. This is the position we find ourselves in every day:

- The doctor is like the professional dancer, familiar with every aspect of the dance floor (by which I mean the consulting room), the language used in the dance and the technical knowledge that underpins it.

- Our patients, on the other hand, vary as much as the celebrities on the show; some are very experienced with perhaps a background in healthcare themselves, or they have become an expert on their own health condition, or they may have simply become very familiar with the dance moves due to the number of consultations they have

3. Larsen, J.-H. and Neighbour, R. (2014) Five cards: a simple guide to beginning the consultation. *British Journal of General Practice,* **64(620):** 150–151.

stacked up over the years. Others feel anxious and out of their comfort zone as soon as they reach the surgery car park, or just don't know where to start when they have to see the doctor.

Just as the professional dancers have to use and adapt their skills as a guide and teacher, so we need to be flexible in our approach to lead both the novice and expert patient through the peculiar interaction that constitutes a consultation. Equally, as the professional dancer manages to keep the celebrity centre stage, so too must we keep the patient at the centre of our particular dance. There are times when one participant will take more of a lead, but throughout the whole consultation it is essential that each player is an active participant. If the doctor starts to do metaphorical pirouettes on their own while the patient stops moving and

> **A doctor who starts to do metaphorical pirouettes while their patient stands and watches is likely to be in trouble!**

Cheese

She had started to think about cheese. It was ridiculous, she knew, but when the doctor mentioned cheese it suddenly reminded her that she had run out and needed to get some for dinner; she was completely out of Cheddar, but maybe a bit of Stilton would add an extra something?

Anne had come to the doctor three weeks earlier; she'd been feeling tired and going to the toilet a lot and was worried that she had developed diabetes like her mother. Now she was back for the blood test results and was relieved to hear there was no sign of the dreaded D. She was feeling better anyway since she'd cut down on caffeine as the doctor had asked her to, and the tiredness just seemed to go on its own. Now the doctor was talking about cholesterol. He'd said it wasn't too bad – didn't he say 4 point something? She was sure that that was quite good, her friend had said hers was 7. Her blood pressure was a bit raised too, but for some reason the doctor was more keen to get her cholesterol down. He'd mentioned something about a risk for something being more than 10%, but Anne hadn't really understood that, and now he was talking about statins; he seemed quite keen that she took them. In passing, he had talked about cheese; he meant her to cut down on it, of course, but all she could think of was that she had forgotten to buy some.

"So, would you like to to give them a try?" asked the doctor.

"I'd rather see how it goes, if that's OK."

The doctor looked a little disappointed, but he didn't push it and they left with a plan to check her blood pressure again in three months. On the way out she decided to leave out the Stilton – she was sure that would please the doctor.

stands back to watch, then the consultation is likely to be in trouble; similarly, if the patient is trying to start the dance and the doctor seems passive and uninterested, then they are failing to guide and lead the patient. Doctor and patient need to move together through the consultation, staying 'in hold' throughout. The skills required to navigate the way through this challenging process are so many and varied that it can be helpful to consider the doctor filling a toolbox with them and bringing this trusted piece of kit with them wherever they go.

Imagining the toolbox

I find it helpful to imagine a physical toolbox filled with tools as real and important as those a plumber would take with them on a job; for the record, mine is red, hinged so that it can expand when I need to delve deep into its recesses, only moderately tidy, and sits in an imaginary space on the floor just to the right of my chair. Every tool is a piece of verbal or non-verbal communication: it may be a single word or utterance like *"Gosh!"* or *"uh-huh"*, a phrase such as *"So, you're not worried about it, you're just fed up with it?"*, or a longer description that might be needed when giving an explanation. What is important is that these are the tools I have developed for my own use since I first started GP training. Many were given to me by my trainer, others have come from reading the classic texts on the consultation or by watching colleagues. All have been tried and tested in the consulting room; ones that didn't work have been thrown out or refined, others tweaked so that they became more effective, and new ones have arisen because, like all healthcare professionals, I just made them up and they seemed to work. What matters is that they feel comfortable in my hand, like the handle of a well-used screwdriver, and they are effective.

There is nothing unusual in this – all doctors will have phrases that they like to use. What matters, though, is to be *intentional* in building up our own toolkit, so that we go through the process of reviewing what works, in order to increase and refine the range of tools available to us. I am sure that I am not alone in having wasted a fruitless afternoon battling with a piece of copper piping, only to call a plumber and watch them fix it in minutes by using the right tool. I still wouldn't be a great plumber even with the right piece of kit, but I would at least have a fighting chance if I were better equipped.

Some of the tools in our toolbox will be in regular everyday use, like a trusted spanner or pair of pliers, while others will be in a lower section of the box, required only on rare occasions. How we choose to greet the patient, the use of silence, sitting forward at the right moment, or phrases like *"tell me…"*, *"you mentioned…"* or *"how do you feel about…?"* all lie at the top of our toolbox, within easy reach for use on multiple occasions every day. On the other hand, a comment like, *"This is actually making me feel a bit overwhelmed, I wonder if that is how it makes you feel?"* might well have its uses, but will lie mostly undisturbed at the bottom of the toolbox, to be retrieved perhaps once a year, but with its place there nonetheless.

What is key about the tools we use is that none of them has a purpose in itself; they are all the means to an end, which are the twin objectives of working out what matters and deciding with the patient what to do about it. Just as there is no point listening with a stethoscope if we then ignore our findings, so there is no value in developing the skills to elicit important information, such as the patient's ideas or concerns, but then failing to use this to help fulfil these objectives. I have frequently observed trainees wrestle with the challenge of this; they have been told that a key task in the consultation is to discover the patient's ideas, concerns and expectations, but if this remains a task to be ticked off then, once complete, it is quickly forgotten. The doctor discovers, for instance, that the patient is worried that their chest pain might be the sign of a heart condition, but they will forget to specifically reassure the patient on this point when they give their explanation. Or the doctor will discover that the patient would really rather not take any pills for their blood pressure, but will stick rigidly to the guidelines anyway and then be surprised by the resistance met when they try to hand over the prescription.

> **If discovering a patient's ICE is thought of as just a task to be ticked off then, once complete, it is quickly forgotten**

Another example of how a classic tool has been subverted in this way is the use of summaries, one of the key checkpoints in the GP consultation described by Neighbour[4]. Trainees have been taught that providing the patient with a summary is a good thing, although they are frequently not so sure about what it is trying to achieve. As a result, they often default to summarising in a way that is familiar to them, as they might on a ward round or when presenting a case. So they simply restate the history with something like:

> *"So, to summarise, you have had this cough for the last week; it started with a fever in the first few days, but this has settled now although you've still got a sore throat and are beginning to lose your voice, is that right?"*

---

4. Neighbour, R. (2015) *The Inner Consultation*, 2nd edition. CRC Press.

The history is restated perfectly, but it achieves nothing and wastes time, possibly even casting doubts in the patient's mind about this doctor's ability to retain facts, since they have only just been told all of this information – can they really be uncertain about it already? What is concerning when GP trainees observe each other consult is that they will often see one of their peers summarise like this and commend them for 'doing a good summary', without asking themselves what it actually achieved. Neighbour does not describe summarising in this way. For Neighbour, summarising is a précis of the doctor's *understanding*, and should be done briefly and periodically to check that the doctor is on the right track, but also to demonstrate understanding to the patient. So it might look something like:

> *"So, you're not worried about your cough, you're more fed up with it and hoping we might be able to do something to help it?"*

Or, perhaps:

> *"So, you can put up with this cough, you just want to make sure it's nothing serious?"*

These phrases are useful tools that crucially help the doctor to work out what matters, and to start looking towards the shared plan. Since more than 30 years have passed since Neighbour wrote *The Inner Consultation*, it is perhaps inevitable that some of his ideas will have become corrupted over time, but perhaps we can reclaim his original intention by incorporating summarising skills into our toolbox. Using the toolbox analogy also removes any sense that the consultation must follow a set pattern. Summarising, for instance, can be used at various stages in the consultation, and was always intended to involve the doctor periodically paraphrasing their understanding, rather than something to be used only once and at a set time point. Neighbour's model structured the consultation as a series of 'checkpoints' with 'Summarising' as the second checkpoint. While this helped with the overall structure, it may also have encouraged a mindset that saw summarising as a single event to take place as the end of the history taking and before coming up with a plan. By considering our consultation skills as tools to achieve an end, rather than tasks to be completed at a set point in the consultation, it is easier to keep the key objectives at the forefront of our minds.

The other advantage of thinking about tools rather than tasks is that we can personalise them. We are not following a consultation model, so much as developing our own bespoke model. We are borrowing from the rich heritage we have from those who have written about the consultation, as well as from those who have trained us, our peers and our own observations on our practice, and both direct and indirect feedback from patients. We should not be content with just making it up as we go along, however, as a sort of lazy, laissez-faire approach to consulting, or use this as a Sinatra-esque excuse to 'do it my way'. We need to evaluate the tools we use and ask simple questions such as 'do they work?' and 'could they be improved?' For instance, we might have been taught to express empathy with a tool like, *"I can see that this has been difficult for you"*. It works, and will be perfect for some situations where a slightly longer statement provides a useful pause, but there will be other occasions where a simple *"Gosh!"* might be more natural; or other times when *"That's tough"* would be more helpful at sending the message of empathy without breaking the patient's flow. We need to build a repertoire of tools in order to fit a range of situations.

> **We are not following a consultation model, so much as developing our own bespoke model**

We evaluate the tools we have chosen by being reflective practitioners, considering carefully the impact of what we do, the immediate response we get from patients and the feedback we receive from them. We need to be prepared to examine ourselves more objectively as well, by direct observation using both simulation and video. Medical students are increasingly exposed to these teaching methods, which is an excellent trend in medical training, but many trainees are still overly self-conscious about the idea of being observed, especially seeing themselves on video – and yet, how else are we to find out what works and what does not? Experienced consulters can lead the way with this, in how we talk about the use of video and simulation, in our own willingness to examine ourselves in the same manner, and in our commitment to the lifelong learning of consultation skills. Just as a chef needs to taste the food before sending it out into the restaurant, so we need to test out what we do whenever we have the opportunity.

Many of the tools that might be used as we explore the *Two Houses* will be discussed in the chapters that follow, where we consider the specific challenges that are posed by particular rooms in each house. At the end of each chapter there will be a table of example tools to consider making use of in that area of the consultation, and the principles that underpin the most effective tools. *Box 3.2* shows some to consider for this chapter.

Box 3.2 Principles and tools to build empathy and keep the dance flowing

Principle for beginning the consultation	If the patient is likely to have prepared an opening gambit, make sure your own opening line doesn't get in the way
Tools to use at the start of the consultation	Initial introduction, then silence to allow the patient to start with their opening gambit *"How can I help today?"* *"What's happening?"* *"Bring me up to speed"* Non-verbal cues for the patient to take the lead: sitting forward, good eye contact, no computer distractions
Principles for encouraging the patient's contribution	Keep your own communication brief but intentional so that it helps to steer the patient and encourage them to keep going Interjections like *"OK"*, *"right"*, etc. can all be helpful, but should be varied and appropriate to what the patient is saying. Saying *"right"* all the time becomes irritating, but also would not be appropriate if someone has just told you that their mother has died! Echoing back, or using phrases like *"you mentioned"* helps to demonstrate good listening
Tools to encourage the patient's contribution	*"Tell me a bit more about the pain"* *"You mentioned your mother"* *"Remind me, have you had this before?"* *"Go on..."* *"And then what happened?"* Where appropriate, echoing the patient's words, e.g. *"it keeps happening..."* or *"quite frightening"* Brief verbal, varied interjections which imply active listening and add meaning, e.g. *"right"*, *"gosh"*, *"OK"*, *"I see"*, *"goodness"* Non-verbal cues that demonstrate active listening, such as sitting forward when appropriate, mirroring body posture, open gestures, hand movements

Principles for keeping the patient with you	Explain your thinking whenever you can so that the patient understands why you are asking the questions you have chosen to ask
	Use of brief summaries of your understanding of what matters to the patient is a really helpful way of making sure you are moving together, and in the right direction
Tools to use when the doctor is taking the lead and needs to keep the patient with them	*"What I'm wondering is whether or not you might have asthma"*
	"We need to be sure that this isn't a kidney infection, so I'll just ask a few questions about that"
	"So you would really like something a bit stronger for the pain?"
	"So your main worry is whether or not this is something you could pass on to your children?"

Chapter 4

Entering the *House of Discovery*

Our homes are intensely personal spaces; we regularly invite people into them, but how we feel about such intrusions depends very much on who it is that is visiting, how they behave, and what they are there for. We would feel very differently about the woman who has come to read the electricity meter, for example, than about the friends we have invited round for dinner. For the former, we would not be surprised if she came unannounced, but would expect to be able to confirm her identity. Once her authenticity is established, she would then have the right to enter the house and go wherever is needed in order to get to the electricity cupboard, but no further; if she were to wander into the lounge and start passing comment on the photographs on the mantelpiece we would probably ask her to leave. Conversely, we might be embarrassed if the path to the electricity meter were completely blocked, but we would not be too worried if the rest of the house were not that tidy. When our friends come round, however, we might well spend time tidying up before they arrive, since we care what they think of us; we might be mortified if they arrived without warning and caught the house in a state, but we would love them to spot the photograph of our children on the mantelpiece and comment on how good they look.

If we consider how we feel personally when someone visits our home, we may be able to understand how patients feel when they allow us into the metaphorical house that constitutes their story, and so learn how best to conduct ourselves when we are afforded that privilege. When we have a visitor we would usually like our house to be reasonably tidy, but might not expect it to be perfect; we hope our visitors won't tread their muddy boots onto our lounge carpet, but don't expect them to be afraid to touch anything for fear of making it dirty. We expect them to wander freely around the main living rooms, but would be somewhat surprised if they made their way up to our bedroom or down into the basement. We hope they will be interested in what they see, that they will like what we like about our house; if they pass comment on a new picture, or the effort we have made in the garden, we will be glad they have taken notice. So too when we tell our story: we want the listener to be interested and respectful. They can ask questions to show their interest, but we would be surprised if these were too personal without good reason; we expect them to find our answers interesting and not to dismiss them or to fire off a stream of unrelated questions. Being a patient involves a degree of vulnerability as you start to let someone in to your story, but just how vulnerable you feel depends on the nature of the problem, and, while the doctor needs to tread with sensitivity, she also needs to act normally. It is remarkable how easily we can forget the value of being normal, which can be especially evident when trainees are starting out in general practice, as they often try too hard.

It is easy to forget the value of being normal: trainees starting out in general practice often try too hard

Being normal

Consider the following start to a consultation:

"Hello Mr Johnson, I'm Dr Abraham, how can I help you today?"

"It's these pains I've been getting in my chest, doctor"

"OK"

"I've had them for a while and they're starting to worry me"

"OK, is it all right if I ask you a few questions about the pains?"

It's not a bad start to the consultation; the doctor has introduced themselves and given space for the patient to say why they are here, and to drop a cue that they are worried about the pains. What, though, is the purpose of the doctor's request for permission to ask more about the pain? It can easily be justified on the grounds that it shows respect, perhaps empathy also, and it has a technical name in the analysis of communication which seems to give it authenticity: it is a statement known as 'signposting', since the doctor is giving a sign that they would like to ask some further questions. But, is it *normal*? If we were down the pub with a friend and they said they were worried about some chest pains, would we ask if it would be OK to ask some questions about it? When is the patient going to say, *"No, it's not OK"*? Are they not there to discuss their chest pains? Asking a question like this is rather like arriving at a friend's house for dinner and then, when they open the door asking, *"Is it OK if I come in?"* or entering the hallway and asking permission to proceed into the kitchen when it is perfectly obvious that this is where they intend us to go.

An alternative way the consultation could have gone would be:

> *"Hello Mr Johnson, I'm Dr Abraham"* (shows Mr Johnson to his seat, waits in silence for him to start)
>
> *"It's these pains I've been getting in my chest, doctor"*
>
> *"Pains?"*
>
> *"Yes, I've had them for a while and they're starting to worry me"*
>
> *"Tell me a bit more"*

This time the dialogue is more natural, and also gives space for the patient's *Opening Gambit*, a concept I have already mentioned that was described by Roger Neighbour[1]. If you have ever sat in the doctor's waiting room you will be very unusual if you have not rehearsed your opening lines (often over and over again, and sometimes even for days before the appointment). This is especially true for a new problem, and so, after introducing herself, Dr Abraham does not need to say *"How can I help you today?"*, since the patient is ready to go and simple silence gives him permission to start the conversation. If you have never started a consultation in silence then I would encourage you to give it a try; usually the patient has started with their opening gambit before they have even sat down. The importance of this pre-

If you have never started a consultation in silence I would encourage you to try it

pared opening gambit came home to me in a new way when we started doing telephone triage. When returning patients' calls they are not expecting you to call at that very moment and, unlike the patient in the waiting room, they are not able to rehearse their opening line as they make their way to your room. For this reason, simply introducing yourself and then using silence does not work well on the telephone; patients usually need a moment to get their thoughts together, and asking how you can help gives them just the time they need.

---

1. Neighbour, R. (2015) *The Inner Consultation*, 2nd edition. CRC Press.

Mr Johnson's first line about his chest pains is followed by the doctor echoing *"Pains?"*, a very natural signal that she has picked up this significant word and invited Mr Johnson to continue, leading to what is probably still part of his rehearsed lines about how the pains are starting to worry him. At this point she pauses, and the doctor's comment, *"Tell me a bit more"* is less an instruction and more an invitation to take his time to continue.

As the consultation proceeds, Dr Abraham might consider the possibility that the chest pains in this young city lawyer could indeed be related to his heart and, knowing that cocaine use is the commonest cause of ischaemic heart disease in young men, might want to ask about this. Now to ask straight out, *"Do you use any drugs?"* would seem abrupt; it is probably not what the patient was expecting and could seem judgemental. This is the equivalent of going into the basement unannounced; we may have good reason to want to go in there, but we need to explain why and ask permission – signposting can be very helpful here and we might try something like:

> *"Can I just check? Sometimes chest pains can be caused by certain street drugs..."*

or

> *"I hope you don't mind me asking, but it's important for me to know if you have ever used any drugs like cocaine."*

The important skill here is to recognise which part of the house we are in, and act both normally and appropriately according to this context.

The surveyor

One of the strangest visitors we have had to our home was when we needed to get our house revalued. A surveyor came at the appointed time, complete with technical equipment such as a laser device for measuring the dimensions of a room, as well as the inevitable clipboard and pen. What was unusual about this particular visitor was that he went systematically through every single room in the house, every bedroom, every toilet, even the garage, the loft space and the garden. In each room he took measurements, recorded notes, occasionally tutted or sucked on his pen, and then moved on to the next room. At no point did he give any clue as to what he was thinking, and when he had finished he said he would submit his report to the mortgage company who would be in touch. We never saw the report ourselves, or even found out what valuation he had made; we were simply told that we could have the mortgage. At the end of the day, the surveyor was professional, he had a job to do and I was happy for him to do it, but there was something oddly unsettling and intrusive about having a stranger look so closely at every aspect of my home in this way, and it wasn't an experience I would want to repeat with any frequency.

The experience with the surveyor was mirrored when I had to have a knee arthroscopy. Various people, from the surgeon to the admitting nurse and the anaesthetist, asked me a series of questions covering every aspect of my medical history without taking much interest in me as a person. Again, this was fine; it was only an arthroscopy and my medical history is rather dull anyway, but what if this series of questions were more personal? What if this were a psychiatric history and it was being taken for the umpteenth time by yet another liaison psychiatric health professional as I lay in a hospital bed after yet another episode of self-harm? How would it feel then? The format for taking a psychiatric history has no more changed since I was at medical school than the medical history model, and it is, necessarily, far more intrusive, routinely requiring questions about sexual history, forensic history, childhood, upbringing and schooling as well as questions about the actual problem the patient has

> **Taking a full psychiatric history is the equivalent of exploring every room in someone's house, including a browse through the photo album, the larder and the underwear drawer**

attended with. It is the equivalent of exploring every room in someone's house, including browsing through the photograph album, the larder and the drawer full of underwear. It has a place, of course, but it is worth stopping to think how familiar a patient with a complex mental health disorder might become with the questions, how they will anticipate what is coming next and will have learnt how to answer them – or not answer them – in the least painful way.

In general practice we have the very great advantage that we don't have to start from scratch every time we see someone; we can build up a picture from the medical record and develop this with every encounter as we form a relationship with the patient, without the need to follow the same pro forma every time we see them. Nevertheless, we are still engaging with the patient in a technical capacity; we are not a friend who has popped round for a cup of tea, but a doctor, and we are expected to do some doctoring! This brings great privileges and permissions that most people would not have, as well as responsibilities to use our technical abilities to the benefit of the patient, to shoulder responsibility and to show leadership.

Thinking like a detective

The increased permissions we are granted mean that, when it is appropriate, we can ask to go into the more private areas of the patient's story; indeed, we may hear something from the patient's life that they have never told anyone before, the equivalent of them retrieving a long-hidden suitcase from the loft and showing us its contents. If we suspect there might be something important hidden in the loft, we are allowed to ask to go and have a look, and when we are shown the suitcase we won't just have a look out of general interest, but will ask searching questions in order to really understand what is inside. This is the art of taking a focused history, and the skills we need to use have more in common with the expert detective than with anyone who takes a clipboard to work. Questions need to be targeted and asked with purpose as we try to understand the problem before us, creating and exploring hypotheses as we consider diagnoses, risks and priorities. Patients expect us to ask such questions, but we need to keep them included in why we are asking them.

The skills a GP needs to use have more in common with the expert detective than with anyone who takes a clipboard to work

Phrases such as, *"I'm wondering about the possibility of…"* or *"Dizziness might be due to low blood pressure, or an inner ear problem; let me ask a few questions to help us decide which it might be"* can be useful tools to keep the patient included in our thinking so that they are engaged with the purpose of the questions we are asking. If our approach comes across as a barrage of seemingly unconnected questions this can leave the patient feeling alienated, while including them in our thinking can empower them and engender trust. As discussed in *Chapter 3*, the doctor needs to stay 'in hold' with the patient in the consultation dance, even at the times when they are taking the lead.

Learning to think like a detective can also enhance the efficiency of the consultation, and a powerful illustration of this targeted, lean approach is how and when we ask about smoking and alcohol consumption. Trainees birthed in the hospital model are used to asking this as part of a social history, meaning the two are indelibly linked together. As a result (particularly in an exam setting where the doctor does not have the notes before them), a patient with depression, appropriately asked about alcohol consumption, will often also be asked if they smoke. Smoking and depression are not strongly linked, if at all, and smokers are probably at their least open to quitting when they are depressed, so asking them about smoking at that moment is not the best opportunity for health promotion, and reminding them of their smoking is unlikely to help how they feel about themselves. Alcohol, on the other hand, is closely linked to depression and patients who are drinking too much are often already aware of the need to cut down and may be open to help and advice in achieving this. Conversely, it makes little sense to ask a patient with asthma about their drinking habits, while smoking, their occupation and any pets at home might be very relevant.

Why does all this matter? Whilst asking about smoking and alcohol together might waste a bit of time, it is hardly a disaster. Why it is important is that it shows that the trainee is not yet thinking like a detective, and is still asking questions because they are meant to be asked, rather than because the trainee really wants to know the answers. This is the transition from asking all the questions you might need and thinking about them later, or presenting them to a senior who will think about them for you, and asking the right questions to achieve that all-important goal: working out what matters.

Narrative questioning

Thinking like a detective is essential when we are trying to make or exclude a diagnosis, and involves a constant process of formulating and testing hypotheses. For example, when we see a patient with a swollen knee we may ask about fever to test the hypothesis of a septic arthritis, or instability if we are considering a cruciate ligament injury. The essential components of such a process are to form hypotheses and ask targeted questions, using the answers to these questions to confirm, change or refine our hypotheses. The same approach can be helpful when it comes to understanding the patient's story as we create a picture of the unique *House of Discovery* we have been asked to visit. Consider the following encounter:

Stress barometer

"I just need an extension of my sick note, I couldn't go to work like this, I wouldn't be able to leave the toilet."

"It has been going on a long time, hasn't it?"

"Yes, I don't know why."

"No. The sample was clear, so it's not an infection, and it's gone on too long for a tummy bug."

"So I'm not infectious?"

"No, and I know that would be a concern for you, working in a school. How have things been at the school?"

"Not great. I've been put in a new class and the teacher I'm with now… she's difficult. It's been stressful."

"How do you think your tummy responds to stress?"

"Hmmm… not great."

Having ruled out infectious causes, the doctor is considering the hypothesis that the patient's ongoing diarrhoea could be caused by stress at work. In this instance, the patient's response that her tummy did not respond well to stress seems to support the hypothesis, and the doctor might enquire more, for instance, by saying, *"That's interesting, how do you think stress affects you?"* The response could have been very different, however; the patient might just as well have said *"Oh, I don't think this is caused by stress. I don't get this sort of problem when I'm stressed."* What is important is that the doctor maintains both a level of curiosity in their questioning so that they can formulate hypotheses, and a willingness to hold these hypotheses lightly, so that they can move on when they do not fit with the patient's story. This narrative approach to the consultation has been well described and I can highly recommend John Launer's wonderful book on narrative-based practice, summed up by the hope-filled subtitle of the book, *conversations inviting change*[2]. Considering the patient's story as analogous to their house works well with a narrative approach, since it reminds us how our understanding (and also the patient's own perception) of their story can build through recurrent visits to their house over a period of weeks, years or even decades.

Chapters 5 to *8* will consider some of the particular challenges we will encounter in the *House of Discovery*, starting with the possibility that the patient may be reluctant to allow us in at all.

2. Launer, J. (2018) *Narrative-Based Practice in Health and Social Care: conversations inviting change*, 2nd edition. Routledge.

Box 4.1 Principles and tools to apply to entering the *House of Discovery*

Principle for beginning the consultation	Consider how to start the consultation so that there is room for the patient's opening gambit
Tools to use on the threshold of the *House of Discovery*	Try using silence, or non-verbals to invite the patient to speak
	Consider a single word in place of silence, such as *"So..."*
	There is nothing wrong with longer opening statements:
	"How can I help?"
	"What are we doing today?"
Principle for keeping a natural flow	Be normal, and ask questions succinctly, guiding the patient with as few words as possible
Tools that can help the doctor gently steer the conversation	*"Tell me about these headaches"*
	"You mentioned your work..."
	Echo key words the patient has used to flag you have heard them, and to invite further comment *"Headaches?"*, *"Frightening?"*
Principles for approaching more private areas in the *House of Discovery*	Ask permission to enter certain areas of the house when it is appropriate; especially where there might be issues of embarrassment, shame or guilt
	Statements can make good questions, especially for more sensitive areas of the house (a point made well by Neighbour)
Tools to use when seeking permission to proceed	*"Can I just ask a couple of safety questions?"*
	"I just need to check a couple of things, if that's OK"
	"Sometimes people find themselves drinking more when they are going through times of stress"
	"It's not uncommon to have thoughts of harming ourselves when we are feeling low"

Chapter 5

Popping the bubble

Engineering

Mark was an engineer and he was used to dealing with problems: find the cause, fix it, problem solved. His back was a problem that kept flaring and it was time to get it fixed. It was obvious that he needed a scan, his friends and family all said the same, and you couldn't fix something if you didn't know what was wrong with it.

"I won't keep you long, doctor, I just need you to sort out a scan for my back." Mark really didn't mean to keep the doctor long; he was sure she was busy enough without him taking up too much of her time.

"OK," came the reply.

It was not the sort of *"OK"* that gave Mark confidence, it was a non-committal *"OK"* and was followed by, *"Tell me a bit more about it and then we can decide if you need a scan."*

Mark felt his jaw tense and the blood vessels rise just a fraction on his temples. One of his friends had warned him about this – *"You might have to fight to get it,"* they'd said. Well if that was how it was going to be…

The role-play scenario of the patient whose opening gambit is to ask for an MRI scan of their back is one of my favourites. Whenever trainees are confronted by it you can see their defences go up in an instant; it is so challenging because it puts the doctor on the back foot in so many ways all at once. For starters, we may find it offends our professional sensibilities; we are the one who went to medical school and spent years as a junior doctor to get to where we are, and we will be the one who decides when a scan is needed and when it is not, thank you very much. Even if we can overcome such a slight to our role, there is the problem that we are being asked to agree to a plan before we know anything about the problem. How can we possibly know if a scan is the right answer before we know anything about the question? In the imagery of the *Two Houses* model, what the patient is effectively doing is meeting us on the threshold of the *House of Discovery* and telling us we don't need to go inside as they know exactly where to go in the other house, so why don't we just go there now?

The scenario usually unfolds with the trainee holding the MRI card tightly to their chest, refusing to make any commitment either way until they have taken a proper history. The patient usually allows some exploration of the history, and even an examination – what other choice do they have? – but with some reluctance. By the time the doctor gets to the point of trying to explain the problem (which, in the role play, is always simply mechanical back pain in which an MRI scan will not be helpful), the patient is not ready to listen, and, sooner or later, will ask *"What about my scan?"* At times the scene can get quite heated, and often the fateful line *"You don't need a scan"* really gets the temperature going – see *Chapter 13* for more on how that word 'need' can utterly derail a consultation.

So how do you tackle a problem like this without getting into a fight? I can only credit my own trainer for this, as he was a true master at it, and it all starts with the very first response to the opening gambit. Instead of asking to hear a bit more, simply say, *"Of course we can arrange a scan."* Trainees usually look at me in horror when I suggest this, and not all will ever feel able to try it out, but a month or two later at least one will say to the group that they had tried it out, and it worked! I learned recently that my now-retired trainer was taught this gem by his own trainer, a lovely reminder of the educational heritage that underpins general practice!

Popping the bubble

Patients sometimes do come to us ready for a fight, but more often they come with a set of beliefs and a clear need to find a way forward for their problem, and if we seem to be obstructive then a fight can follow. From the outset, the questions that are likely to be in their mind are: *Am I going to be listened to? Will I be taken seriously, or just fobbed off?* Sometimes there is a genuine belief that the best way to save the doctor time is a quick appointment with the desired outcome achieved with as little fuss as possible, and they have not thought that the doctor must take clinical responsibility for the plan. These consultations usually revolve around a problem that the patient is keen to get solved, and do tend to start with a higher degree of tension than most; the question is whether this tension will start to escalate or dissipate. If we can pop the bubble of tension before

If we can pop the bubble of tension before it gets going then we have the best chance of avoiding conflict

it gets going then we have the best chance of avoiding conflict, and we are more likely to achieve a shared understanding of the problem.

What happens if we say at the outset that we can do the scan? The first thing is that the tension usually drops and the patient is happy to tell us more about the problem; we are invited into the *House of Discovery* and allowed to look around. We have not promised to do a scan, but what we have done is say to them that there is a room in the house next door marked 'MRI scans', that we know how to get there and that we *will* visit it with them. This is often enough; as we show we are listening to the patient, so they are more likely to listen to us. There are then three possible outcomes:

1. We decide they do indeed need an MRI scan; we can agree with them, arrange the scan and everyone leaves happy.
2. It is clear that a scan will not add much, but we have been able to develop a shared understanding with the patient and they are happy to accept a different way forward.
3. It is clear that a scan will not add much, but the patient remains insistent and demands that we refer them for one.

Outcome 2 can often be successfully negotiated once the bubble has been popped and the doctor and patient are able to truly listen to each other. For example, the patient may believe that scans always give an answer, but learning that scans are disappointingly uninformative in mechanical back pain may make them more open to alternative solutions such as physiotherapy. This outcome means that we have found, and been able to navigate around, an *Empty* or *Locked Room*, which will be explained in more detail in *Chapter 13*.

In my experience Outcome 3 is very rare, and if it were to happen, then being more confrontational or obstructive at the beginning is only likely to make things worse; if someone is that determined, we are unlikely to come to a shared understanding however we play things.

Of course, you cannot take this approach with every demand a patient makes. A patient once presented me with an opening request to prescribe him with testosterone because when he was given some by his mates at the gym it improved his performance! Clearly, if the request is unethical, impossible or illegal we should not say that we can do it. I am certainly wary of taking this approach with requests for controlled drugs, for instance, but even here we can still say that we can talk about it rather than just ignoring the request.

Finding alternative solutions to the problem

Overcoming a blockage

"I won't take much of your time, doctor, I just need you to refer me to an Ear Nose and Whatever doctor."

"Sure, we can do that. What's going on?"

"It's my nose. Always blocked. I'm sure I've got a polyp."

"That's annoying. How long's it been happening?"

Dr Mittal took her time to find out more. She was encouraged that she was allowed to; when he came in he was in such a hurry to get the referral and leave that she thought he wouldn't even sit down. The symptoms certainly fitted with nasal allergy, and could well be a polyp; his friend had had the same problem for months and only eventually got it removed.

"You're absolutely right that this could be a polyp," she said, *"and we could certainly refer you to a specialist. The first thing they always do for polyps, though, is to see if they will shrink back with a steroid nasal spray, and I'm wondering if we shouldn't just start that rather than waste your time with a referral at this stage if that's all they would do."*

He didn't seem too opposed to this idea, so she went on. *"The spray doesn't work straight away, but if we did a trial for the next 6–8 weeks, then if it wasn't any better you could let me know and we could do the referral then. We'd be one step ahead as we'd have already done the first thing they always do."*

Dr Mittal's patient left, finding himself surprised by how happy he felt with the plan.

An early demand for a particular outcome is usually a strong indicator that the patient is looking for a solution to their problem

An early demand for a particular outcome is usually a strong indicator that the patient is looking for a solution to their problem and not just better understanding (see *Chapter 9, A house with two wings*, for more on this subject). Once the tension bubble has been popped, by agreeing to the possibility of the solution they have hit upon, the doctor will be given more space to work out whether or not that is indeed the best solution to their problem. In the example of the nasal polyp, the desire for a referral was based on the assumption that a physical polyp needed physical removal, backed up by the experience of a friend who had needed to have an operation for their own polyp. The desired outcome, however, was not to have surgery, but to have relief from the symptoms. Once it is explained that a spray may be just as effective – and even more so the fact that they could wait for an appointment only to be told the same thing – the desire for a referral can recede. Combine this with a plan to refer in the future, and with a clear timescale, and the patient can be surprisingly happy with the outcome, even if it was not what they expected when they walked in.

Popping the angry bubble

I will show my age here, but when I was first a student, cash machines still gave out £5 notes. I remember this distinctly because my usual withdrawal was just that, £5, and it always felt a bit rash to withdraw £10 in one go! Therefore when my bank made a charge on my account of £10, this was a significant dent in my troubled finances, and, since I was sure the charge was unjust, I contacted the bank with fierce determination to get my money back. I remember it well – I had rehearsed my reasoning, my opening gambit and every counterargument; I was ready to fight. The call lasted only a few minutes as the person I spoke to quickly told me I was right, how sorry they were and of course they would refund the money straight away. I was pleased, of course, but in a strange way my bubble of self-righteous injustice had been popped so quickly and so effectively that I felt slightly deflated; I was ready for a fight, but it is hard to fight someone when they won't fight back!

Exactly the same principle holds true when we have an angry patient, or someone making a complaint. Tension levels can be extremely high when the consultation starts with anger, and the initial response of the doctor can be crucial in determining the outcome. If we can acknowledge quickly *and sincerely* that we understand the reason for the anger, and accompany this with a meaningful apology, this can be a remarkably effective way to defuse tension, sometimes with dramatic and very rewarding results. The crucial word here is 'sincerely', as an insincere apology will usually make things worse. Sincerity, or a lack of it, is communicated in every aspect of what we say and do. It includes

> **The crucial word is 'sincerely', as an insincere apology will usually make things worse**

non-verbal communication such as the use of eye contact and open body language as well as the tone and pitch of our voice. When we do start to speak, we should pick our words carefully; even something like, *"I am so sorry this has happened"* is more sincere than, *"I'm sorry this has made you angry"*, since the latter leaves an implication that the person's choice to become angry is what we are sorry about, rather than the circumstances that led to the anger.

Doctors often worry about admitting responsibility when they apologise, but the idea that saying sorry increases the chance of litigation is a myth that must be dispelled. Of course we should not speak badly of colleagues who are not there to defend themselves, but an unqualified apology is so unlikely to increase the chance of a complaint escalating that I would suggest it can only ever be helpful, and in the vast majority of cases there will be some justification for it once the facts are fully understood; people rarely become angry for no reason at all. Of course, there is much more to dealing with a complaint than simply popping the angry bubble, and helping the angry patient will be covered in more detail as a topic for one of the *Two Houses* guides in *Chapter 15*.

A pop in time

Whether dealing with an angry patient, a demand for a home visit or insistence on a referral, a common theme to all these consultations is that the window of opportunity to pop the bubble is brief, and usually happens very early on. If this opportunity is missed then defusing the tension becomes steadily more difficult as doctor and patient take up increasingly separate positions; as the old proverb says, *'a stitch in time saves nine'*. The challenge this presents is that the doctor has to pop the bubble before having all the facts, which appears to involve an element of risk, even though it is probably the least risky strategy to take! If you remain sceptical, I can't blame you, but why not find out for yourself, take a risk and give it a go?

> **The window of opportunity to pop the bubble is brief, and usually happens very early on**

Box 5.1 Principles and tools for popping the bubble

Principle	Wherever you can, acknowledge the validity of the request as a means of popping the bubble
Tools to pop the bubble	*"Of course we can arrange a visit, what's the problem?"* *"We can certainly arrange a referral; tell me what's happening"* *"That sounds tough – we can certainly talk about painkillers"*
Principle	If the initial request isn't the best way forward, try to achieve a shared understanding
Tools for achieving a shared understanding	*"We could certainly refer you to a dermatologist now, but I know which creams they always recommend first, and I wonder if it would be better if we did that to start with and then, if they aren't working, we'd be one step further on when we do refer you"* *"My worry about a scan is that often they are very disappointing and don't tell us anything we don't already know, but I think a physiotherapist would really be able to help you right now"* *"We definitely need to see you and I realise it's not easy for you to get here, but it would really help us if you could come down to the surgery, and we would be able to see you more quickly"*
Principle for popping the angry bubble	Apologise quickly and sincerely, agree with the patient where you can
Tools for dealing with anger	*"I am so sorry this has happened"* *"I'm really sorry that something has gone wrong – tell me what's happened"* *"It's very understandable that this has made you want to complain"*

Chapter 6

Exploring the basement

According to official Government statistics, compiled by the Gambling Commission in 2016, 0.7% of people in the UK aged 16 and over are classified as 'problem gamblers'[1]. For our practice, therefore, with close to 9000 patients in this age range, we should expect to have over 60 problem gamblers. We have a reasonably average demographic and so our disease prevalence figures are rarely far removed from national averages; thus it is reasonable to assume that we must have at least 40 or 50. Why then, can I not think of any patient who is a problem gambler? Not a single one. I have been in the practice for eighteen years and I don't find it difficult to recall patients; I can easily bring to mind a number who have alcohol or drug addiction, many who have been suicidal over the years, and several who have been dependent on food banks or been malnourished as they couldn't afford to eat. It is not hard to remember some who have been in and out of prison – some who are still inside – and it is easy to think of patients I have cared for who have had all manner of cancers, unusual neurological conditions or textbook endocrine disorders. The national prevalence of 0.7% is the same as that of rheumatoid arthritis – and which GP doesn't have patients with this? And yet, I cannot think of a single problem gambler.

What is happening here? In part it is my failings as a doctor – I have not been good at asking about gambling; indeed, it has only even occurred to me that I *should* ask about it in the last two to three years. No doubt, also, there is a failing in my medical education; I was taught to take a social history, but this focused on factors such as smoking, alcohol and drug use as well as occupational history (with the emphasis on occupational disease, not financial wellbeing) as well as who else was at home, including pets if I wanted to be thorough. I was never taught to take a financial history, let alone ask about gambling. Sadly, a quick internet search on how to take a medical history suggests nothing has changed here. Maybe we are just too British to ask about money!

---

1. The Gambling Commission (2016) *Gambling Participation and Problem Gambling*. Available at: bit.ly/2SlzTVk (accessed February 2020).

Whatever the failings on my part, however, the invisibility of my problem gambling patients has convinced me that there are parts of the *House of Discovery* that our patients are very good at keeping hidden. Consultations almost never start with *"I need help with my gambling"*, nor do patients mention it with their hand on the door as they are about to leave. Maybe they don't see it as a health problem, although its health consequences can be devastating. More likely we do see these patients, or their partners, parents or children, all affected by the impact of gambling; yet they pass through our doors repeatedly with the secret of gambling securely stored away in the basement of their lives, a rug thrown innocuously over the trapdoor that leads down into this part of their story, so that we don't even suspect its presence.

> **There are parts of the *House of Discovery* that our patients are very good at keeping hidden**

Recognising the basement

Just who she was

Sasha liked this doctor; she had seen him a few times and he always seemed to listen. They usually talked about her anxiety and he often had a helpful tip to share; just talking about it seemed to help. He'd wanted her to think about medication, of course, but she hadn't liked to go that way – weight gain and all that; he didn't seem to mind.

They'd never talked about food.

It wasn't that she would refuse to talk about it, or would be annoyed if he'd asked; she was just so used to keeping it private. The clothes she wore didn't seem baggy or like she was trying to hide something any more, they were just her *look*; eating on her own was just something she did – her flatmates knew that she liked her own company.

So when she saw the doctor she didn't even think to talk about food; how she ate was something that helped her manage her anxiety, after all, not the cause of it. It wasn't like keeping a secret; it was just who she was.

The first requirement for approaching the basement is to recognise its existence. We can consider it as a room (or even a suite of rooms) in the *House of Discovery* that we all have and that contains the things we like to keep hidden. This is no trendy refurbished basement complete with a cinema or well-stocked wine cellar, but a musty, cluttered and dingy space we don't like to think about, and it certainly isn't a room for visitors.

Simply recognising that there might be something important in the basement is a great start, but we then need to consider what we might find there. Some of this is very familiar to the medical profession, and patients are equally used to us enquiring about it; alcohol, for instance, commonly finds its way into the basement, but is something doctors are expected to ask about. We play an uneasy game where patients expect us to double the amount they admit to and they try to guess whether they should be truthful, or really ought to lie and halve the amount just so we get the maths right! Similarly, smoking, drug use and suicidal ideation are aspects of the basement that as doctors we know we need to ask about, but even in this familiar territory we encounter different challenges; the skills required to enquire about thoughts of self-harm are clearly more complex than those needed to take a smoking history. We might consider the basement as having degrees of depth, with social and cultural factors involving secrecy, embarrassment and shame pushing problems deeper into its shadows.

There can be no exhaustive list of what we might find in the basement, but it is worth considering the sort of issues that might be hidden within its walls. There are two key aspects that lead to something finding its way into the basement: first, a degree of reluctance on the part of the patient to mention it, and secondly, the fact that the issue could be important for their health. Here is some of what we might find when we venture into the basement:

- Smoking
- Alcohol and drug misuse
- Self-harm, such as through cutting, or suicidal thoughts
- Financial problems and debt
- Gambling
- Domestic abuse
- Family shame
- Sexual problems, including issues of sexuality and gender
- Eating disorders
- Symptoms of obsessive–compulsive disorder (OCD)
- Past traumas, whether childhood abuse, or an intense event that might lead to post-traumatic stress disorder
- Other complex issues such as the impact of war and conflict, modern slavery, prostitution and radicalisation, although these are highly specialised and so won't be expanded upon here.

Of course, we should not expect that these issues are always to be found in the basement – issues of sexual orientation and gender, for instance, have increasingly found their way out of the basement as our society, thankfully, no longer sees these as issues of shame to be hidden away. However, shame is a highly personal and sociocultural issue and what matters is what the patient finds shameful enough to have hidden away, not what we might judge to be shameful. What ties all these issues together is that it is easy to conduct an otherwise very effective consultation without uncovering them, despite their importance. OCD is a case in point here; it never ceases to surprise me how easy it is to talk in depth about a patient's anxiety, even over several consultations, and only find out very late in the day that they have complex, even life-controlling symptoms of OCD. I wonder how many patients of mine are yet to reveal it to me, and how many I have neglected to ask.

Navigating the basement

There are questions we should always ask ourselves when we are thinking of the basement, and we will consider them in turn.

Should we ask for permission to enter?

We have already considered how requesting permission to ask straightforward questions (for instance, by saying *"Is it OK if I ask a few questions about your chest pain?"*) can be both a waste of time and confusing for the patient. Entering the basement, however, is not like going into the hallway or the kitchen. If we are visiting a friend's house, we are unlikely to just wander down there; if there is a good reason to want to see their basement, we are at least likely to say something like *"Ooh, can I have a look?"*. So too for the virtual basement of the patient's story. Most of the time it will be important to ask for permission, or give a signpost that we would like to ask about something more sensitive. A simple question like *"Can I just ask how much alcohol you drink?"* may suffice, or a signpost such as *"Before we decide what we might do next, I'd just like to ask a couple of safety questions if that's OK"*, which might then lead to questions about alcohol and self-harm.

Is it necessary to enter the basement?

We have to respect that we are entering someone else's story when we ask them questions, and since the basement is the most secret part of their story, it clearly must be necessary and proportionate to their problem that we ask to be allowed access. It would be highly inappropriate, for instance, to enquire about someone's sexuality if all they have come about is a problem with earwax, or to ask if someone is in debt just because their T-shirt is a bit scruffy! Even when the nature of the problem does justify asking further questions, we need to think carefully. For something that could reveal deep wounds, such as abuse for instance, there still needs to be consideration as to whether or not this is the right time and place to ask such questions. Have we built sufficient rapport and trust to be the one asking? Who else is in the room that might not have a right to hear the answers? Is the person just too vulnerable right now to tackle this? Neither, on the other hand, should we allow such concerns to prevent us from asking difficult questions when the time is right.

> We have to respect that we are entering someone else's story, and the basement is the most secret part of that story

How should we phrase the question?

In fact, do we even need to ask a question? In *The Inner Consultation*[2], Roger Neighbour talks about the value of statements as a substitute for a question in these circumstances. Statements like:

> *"Sometimes people have a compulsion to do something repeatedly to avoid feeling anxious"*

or

> *"Sometimes when people are stressed they find themselves drinking more alcohol"*

can be very effective ways of exploring the basement without putting the person on the spot. It may also allow for more honesty. If the patient replies *"Yes, I think I am drinking more than I usually do"* they have already admitted that there may be an issue, and they may then give a more honest answer

---

2. Neighbour, R. (2015) *The Inner Consultation*, 2nd edition. CRC Press.

when asked to quantify their drinking than if they are asked from the start, *"How much are you drinking?"* Explaining our own thinking can also be helpful, for instance, *"When I hear a story like this it makes me wonder about past abuse"* might be kinder, and more effective, than the direct equivalent *"Have you ever been abused?"*

Direct questions can also be very effective, especially when they are asked in an open way. Something like, *"Can you tell me how you feel about food and eating?"* might be more fruitful than, *"Do you think you have an eating disorder?"*. Similarly, a general enquiry about an aspect of someone's life can be very helpful as an opening into a sensitive area, without being directly threatening, such as, *"How were things for you, growing up?"* or *"How are things at home?"*.

Things to remember

Different rooms in the *House of Discovery* bring with them different rules of engagement, and there are some important rules to remember when considering the basement:

1. **Always respect the patient's right to deny access**
   Of course, this applies to all aspects of the house, but we need to be especially mindful of it in the basement. Even something as simple as trying to quantify someone's alcohol consumption can feel like a violation of their privacy if done clumsily, and there is an even greater risk when enquiring about abuse, self-harm or someone's relationship with food.

2. **Allow time**
   If there is a clear 'no' to an enquiry then we can quickly move on, but where an issue is identified, it will take time to explore. For instance, if someone does have financial worries, what is the extent of them? Where have they come from? Is there debt? What about gambling? Or uncontrolled spending? Is this something temporary with a clear way out, or is the person in such a sea of debt that they are looking at insolvency? Have they sought advice? All these questions will need to be asked in the context of someone who is likely to be distressed and so it is not like rattling through questions relating to a cough or a sore knee. For emotionally charged issues like abuse, it may be too much to expect to explore in one consultation; there is only so much we have time for, but, even more importantly, there is only so much a patient can take in one go.

3. **Don't be surprised if the patient is in denial**

   When we hide things away in the basement, we hide them from ourselves as well as others, and so what may appear to the doctor to be obvious domestic abuse, a very abnormal relationship with food and eating, or unusual rituals that need to be performed in order to be able to leave the house in the morning, may have become so normalised that the patient does not recognise them for what they are. We need to be careful that we don't leave the patient behind, and understand if they take a while to catch up with us, even if this takes several consultations, or even years.

4. **Tie certain questions together in your mind**

   When we are taught how to take a medical history, smoking and alcohol are always tied together as inseparable twins in the social history, even though there are very few problems where they are both directly relevant. When it comes to exploring the basement it is worth making new partnerships that cannot be thought of on their own. The most useful is self-harm and alcohol. There are plenty of occasions where it is reasonable to ask about alcohol consumption and not self-harm, but if we need to ask about self-harm, we will also always want to ask about alcohol. They are both vital safety questions to ask with the majority of mental health problems and work well as a pair. Similarly, we should get into the habit of asking about debt whenever someone mentions financial worries, and, where there is debt, to ask about gambling. The links between anxiety and OCD or an eating disorder are less strong, but we should at least have them loosely linked in our minds so that we are more likely to remember these important issues when helping an anxious patient; maybe we should always ask about them with anxiety, or is that going too far?

5. **Use confidence to help relieve the patient's embarrassment**

   Patients may be fine exploring the basement, but some will feel shame or embarrassment and the doctor can help to reduce these feelings by remaining respectful, but also confident in a way that normalises having a conversation about the issues that are being encountered. If the doctor is embarrassed, shocked or offended by what they find in the basement then this does not bode well for the patient, whereas it can be enormously therapeutic if the patient can trust that their problems are something we are not unused to, nor shocked by, nor afraid of.

> **If the doctor is embarrassed, shocked or offended by what they find in the basement this does not bode well for the patient**

Box 6.1 Principles and tools to apply to the basement

Principle	Ask for permission to enter, or signpost where you are heading
Tools for asking permission to enter the basement	*"I'd just like to ask a couple of important questions if that's OK"* *"One thing that's important to ask – have you ever used street drugs?"*
Principle	Statements make good questions
Tools for asking questions with statements	*"Sometimes food can become a big issue when we are stressed"* *"It's not uncommon to have thoughts of harming yourself"* *"Sometimes feelings like this can start after a very traumatic event"* *"I'm worried that you might be being abused"*
Principle	Don't be afraid to ask the difficult questions
Tools for asking difficult questions	*"How are things in your marriage?"* *"Is there anything in your past you think might be affecting you now?"* *"Are you in debt?"*

Chapter 7

Finding dry rot

The heart of the matter

Anne was glad the doctor was running on time; she had a busy day planned and had managed to squeeze in the appointment between dropping her grandson off at school and picking her father up for a hospital appointment; she had enough time, but her father always hated the idea that he might be late and she didn't want to stress him. She had nearly cancelled; the pain had only been there a week or so and was bound to go away on its own, but she felt she *ought* to get it checked, and so here she was. Maybe he'd give her something for it.

"So, you say that this pain comes when you walk up a hill, but goes away quickly when you stop?"

"Yes." That was good, wasn't it? That the pain didn't last?

From the look of concern on the doctor's face, he didn't seem to agree that this was good.

"I'm a bit worried that this pain might be coming from your heart."

Her heart? But she'd always had a good heart; wasn't it men that got heart problems? And smokers?

And anyway, she really didn't have time to have a problem with her heart.

When I was a young child my parents decided to rework the ground floor of our house. It wasn't a large project, but with three children and the whole of the upstairs given over to lodgers it would help to make space for us all. Money was tight, and so when the work started and the builders found dry rot, it was something of a disaster. I was too young to know much about it, or to understand the strain it put on our finances, but as I grew up, dry rot became symbolic as the worst thing that could happen to a house. There was something malign in the idea that the core of your home could be eaten away without you knowing, and that one day you might innocently lift up a carpet and unearth a scene of devastation; my mother was always afraid that it would strike again. As an adult, the logical way to defend afraid that it would strike again. As an adult, the logical way to defend against such an eventuality in my own home would be to learn about the causes of dry rot and find ways to protect my house from being affected; my slightly more nuanced approach, however, has been to shy away from reading anything whatsoever about dry rot, avoid looking at horrible pictures of what it can do and hope it never happens – so far this strategy is working well!

When we are invited into a patient's *House of Discovery*, we are not merely visitors, come to admire the décor, but technicians equipped with expert knowledge and specialist equipment, ready to evaluate, investigate and diagnose their problem. Often, this is straightforward, with patient and doctor expecting a similar diagnosis for which there is a simple management plan. A far greater challenge is where the diagnosis is more significant or the outlook more uncertain, and when this comes as a shock to the patient, the challenge is greater still. We have lifted the carpet and found dry rot.

> **Where a diagnosis is significant, or the outlook uncertain, we have lifted the carpet and found dry rot**

Traditionally, this is called *breaking bad news*, and it is a good term as it places the emphasis on how to break the news, which is what matters in the end. I have wrestled with describing this process as *finding dry rot* – is it disrespectful? Is it too dramatic? Too unpleasant? It is certainly not the sort of professional term we would expect doctors to be using; but maybe that is the problem with some of the terms we use, that they can be too professional sometimes, too clinical, too lacking in emotion.

I wrote a blog a while ago on our practice website, entitled *Who's Afraid of the Big Bad C?*[1] The piece was about how, for many people, the worst thing about being diagnosed with cancer was not dying from it – we all have to die of something – but being *diagnosed* with it and having to do the *'cancer thing'*; the surgery, radiotherapy, chemotherapy; the telling people and having them talk about us; the comments on how we were coping; the awkward conversations with people who don't know what to say. The point I was raising was that in our drive to stop people from dying of cancer, by virtue of screening and ever-earlier diagnosis, we were exposing far more people to the actual process of being diagnosed with cancer, which in itself is a massive, life-changing event.

---

1. Brunet, M. (2012) *Who's Afraid of the Big Bad C?* The Binscombe Doctor Blog. Available at: bit.ly/2GTt9J8 (accessed February 2020)

One of my patients left the following comment after reading the blog:

> Oh dear! That word. That awful word. I'm afraid I had to skip
> through your article, scanning quickly so as not to absorb
> all you said. It always affects me this way. Just thinking or
> reading about C makes me feel sick and my legs start jumping
> up and down. I was glad when I reached the end of the article.
> Phew! I've escaped cancer again. What a relief. Daft? Nope,
> just plain scared!

There is no doubt that, for this patient, to tell him that he had cancer would not just be a matter of breaking bad news, it would have all the horror and unpleasantness of finding dry rot, and more on top, since it is his body we would be talking about and not just his home. Of course, another patient will hardly bat an eyelid when we explain they might have cancer, but perhaps associating bad news with a degree of abhorrence is helpful for the doctor to empathise with how the patient might be feeling. When we think of ourselves in the patient's house having found signs of dry rot, we might consider that we are standing next to them, looking at the damaged floorboards together. This togetherness is important when tackling a serious problem like this, whereas the concept of breaking bad news can leave an image of the doctor holding the bad news, passing it to the patient, however carefully, and leaving them to it. Of course, the patient is the one left with the problem whatever we may call this process, but the sense that the doctor will journey with them regardless of what the future holds is one of the most important aspects of primary care, and can be powerfully therapeutic.

> **The sense that the doctor will journey with the patient regardless of what the future holds is one of the most important aspects of primary care**

Anticipating dry rot

One of the key aspects of the consultation is that the doctor needs to do some doctoring! As described in *Chapter 4*, we need to think like a detective and, where we can, use our technical skills to bring the problem to a diagnosis. Alongside such thinking, we also need to anticipate the seriousness of the problem, and the likely response of the patient sitting in front of us.

In an instant

Dr Gupta wasn't quite sure why she had asked if the child could provide a urine sample, but she often found that the time the machine took to analyse the results gave her invaluable thinking space. She wasn't sure what was going on with this five-year-old, but her instinct told her that he wasn't well. As soon as she dipped the stick in the urine, her thinking space took a dramatic turn as she saw the glucose strip rapidly turn dark brown.

Diabetes.

In a moment she was going to have to turn this child's world, and that of his parents, upside down. It was bizarre how this life-changing diagnosis was made in an instant; no need for a confirmatory test; no doubt that he needed to go to hospital; no changing the fact that he would need insulin... forever.

Just as patients rehearse their opening gambit in the waiting room and steel themselves before they are called, so Dr Gupta found herself rehearsing how to break this news; she took a deep breath as she went back into her consulting room.

Sometimes finding dry rot is as dramatic as pulling back the carpet and suddenly revealing the problem, as in the case of dipping the urine of a child with previously undiagnosed diabetes – there are few life-changing diagnoses that can be made with such certainty and such speed. At other times, the level of concern rises more gradually. It may be a worrying symptom or a concerning examination finding that needs to be investigated, a blood test that suggests more investigations are warranted, or symptoms that are not resolving in the anticipated time frame. The skill of the doctor is to keep the patient with them at all times; we don't want to leave them behind, failing to grasp the seriousness of the situation, but neither should we alarm them by listing every possible, fearful diagnosis. It is interesting how often the attempt of the medical profession to rule out serious, but unlikely, diagnoses is interpreted by patients and their families as having a *'cancer scare'* or *'they think there's something wrong with her heart'*.

Principles to use when navigating dry rot

There is a significant body of work on breaking bad news in the medical literature. However, as I have mentioned before, this book is not an academic work or a review of the literature, but a collection of my own thoughts and experience which you can incorporate into your own practice where you find them helpful.

1. Discover the patient's level of concern

Of course, this goes back to ICE and exploring the patient's concerns, but what really matters here is not their specific concern, but understanding the *level* of concern. If a patient has an exact concern – *"I'm worried I might have bowel cancer, doctor"* – then that is always helpful to elicit. However, as we have previously discussed, patients frequently don't have an exact concern that they can name. What *all* patients have, though, is a level of concern, which can vary from having no concern at all to being convinced that they are dying. Once we have discovered this – either by careful observation of cues or direct enquiry – we know the patient's starting point and where we have to work from.

> **Once we have discovered the patient's level of concern, we know their starting point and where we have to work from**

2. Start to bridge the gap between the patient's level of concern and your own

When doctor and patient have very different levels of concern, the process of breaking bad news is much more challenging, and steps need to be taken to bridge that gap. In the example with Anne at the start of the chapter, there was a clear gulf between Anne's very low level of concern and the doctor's assessment that she might have angina. To go straight to a management plan of a referral to the chest pain clinic, blood tests, aspirin and a GTN spray would be utterly bewildering for her without first trying to bridge this gap. Overtly expressing our level of concern, using words like 'concern' and 'worry' can be a helpful starting point:

> *"I'm always concerned when someone tells me they have pain that comes and goes with exertion"*

> *"I do worry a bit when I hear that food gets stuck"*

Actively using the word 'serious' or 'seriously' can also be a way of raising concern without causing alarm:

> *"We do take it seriously when someone loses weight without trying"*

Always avoid the word 'sinister', though; *"We need to rule out anything sinister"* is likely to not only bring the patient up to our level of concern, but fling them way beyond it!

Sometimes we need to bring the patient down to a lower level of concern if actually they are more worried than they need to be. That is easiest when we can completely reassure them that all is well, but requires more care when there remains uncertainty:

> *"I do think we should check this out in the breast clinic, but I will be expecting them to find that there is nothing serious here."*

3. Leave space

Probably the most important principle of all is to pause and use silence when you break bad news. Words like, *"I am worried this might be cancer"* or *"I think you need to go into hospital"* need some time to sink in before the patient is ready to hear anything more. It can be tempting to rush on and give some good news in order to balance the bad – the good prognosis for the cancer or the fact that the hospital stay should be short, for instance – but this is a temptation that must be resisted. Let the bad news sink in and give time for the patient to respond first, and then they will be ready to hear the better news.

> **The most important principle of all is to pause and use silence when you break bad news**

4. Don't be afraid to name it

I remember observing a trainee in a simulation session. The scenario was a man with back pain returning to discuss blood results. His prostate-specific antigen test was over 100, which meant an unequivocal diagnosis of prostate cancer and the very high probability of metastatic spread to the spine. This very able trainee conducted a skilled, empathetic and medically correct consultation; she paused as she gave the bad news that the test was abnormal and the situation was serious, and explained the need for an urgent referral. It was high quality in every way except that at no point did she use the word 'cancer'.

In the feedback session after she had finished, we explored why she had shied away from telling this man that he had cancer. What emerged was that it was due to the finality of being the one to give him the diagnosis. As a junior doctor she had never been the one to both make the diagnosis and give the news; previously a more senior doctor, or a team of doctors, had concluded the diagnosis and if she was the one to give the bad news, she never carried the responsibility for it on her own. In general practice it is easy to forget how unusual it is for young doctors to do this; she knew 100% that he had cancer, but the nagging *"what if I'm wrong?"* doubt in her head stopped her saying the word.

Some patients will help us out by using the word 'cancer' themselves, but others will not; they may not have thought of it, or they may be thinking of nothing else, but unable to say the word. Either way, there are times when the doctor needs to show leadership and just name it. This might be when breaking the bad news, or in explaining what we are testing for, or what we need to consider if symptoms don't settle. For instance, to ask someone to come back with a repeat urine *"to check the blood has cleared"* is one thing, but if we want the patient to grasp the importance of the repeat test then we may need to add sensitively that bladder cancer is something we might need to consider if the blood doesn't clear.

5. Allow the time that you will need

When we know we have bad news to give, it will take time, and we need to plan for this. There will be the delivery of the bad news itself, handling the emotional reaction to the news and then the high likelihood of a complex plan to negotiate, information to pass on and questions to answer. This is most relevant for trainees sitting the CSA exam – at least in real practice we can just run late if we get this wrong, but in the exam setting the bell may ring and the patient leaves, taking half the marks for that scenario with them since important points were never covered. Usually the signs that time will be needed are there from the beginning – an abnormal test result or a worrying symptom in the opening salvos – yet, time and again, trainees seem to panic in the knowledge that they have bad news to break, dilly-dallying in the history while they build up courage, only to find themselves pitifully short of time once they finally tackle the real issue.

6. Remember that, sometimes, bad news is good news, and good news can be bad

There is a lot to be said for certainty, and often a diagnosis, even a serious one, is easier to deal with than the uncertainty of not understanding what is wrong with you. Conversely, apparently good news can be difficult to

Sifting the wheat from the chaff

Ravi shifted in his seat as the doctor shuffled the pieces of paper on the desk.

"I've got your test results," she began. *"And we have found the cause of your symptoms."* She paused. *"It is quite serious…"*

Ravi's heart skipped a beat and nearly stopped at the same time; she'd found the cause, what did she mean by serious?

"Your tests show you have probably got coeliac disease."

From the look on her face, she obviously thought this was something he might take badly, but Ravi felt like a weight had been taken off him. Coeliac disease – that was serious, and he didn't know much about it, but he knew there was something you could do about it.

"I was so worried you were going to say there was nothing wrong with me."

> **Where the patient is looking for a solution, reassurance may come across as a denial of their problem**

deal with. Avril Danczak[2] wrote an excellent essay in the *BMJ* on the subject of breaking good news and how telling someone how great it is that their tests are all normal can be hugely problematic. Where the patient is looking for a solution (see *Chapter 9* for more on this), reassurance may not only be unhelpful, but could come across as a denial of their problem. Acknowledging this when giving the results can be helpful:

> *"Your blood tests are normal, which is reassuring, but it obviously doesn't give us any answers."*

Conclusions

Finding 'dry rot' and helping the patient to navigate their way through it can be one of the greatest challenges a doctor will face. It requires a high level of deductive reasoning to determine the seriousness of the situation, which must be accompanied by a sensitivity to the verbal and non-verbal cues from the patient. The doctor must remain attentive to what the patient is thinking and feeling; are they anticipating something serious? Have they been able to express themselves and are they feeling that their

---

2. Danczak, A. (2018) Breaking good news: an essential skill for avoiding too much medicine? *BMJ*, **362**: k3843.

story has been heard? Are they able to understand the situation? Do they need more time to adjust, or are they so worried they just want to get on to a plan as quickly as possible? There is no doubt that holding this dual responsibility of listening to the patient's story while also bringing clinical expertise and reasoning to the problem requires a great deal of skill, but it can also be one of the most rewarding aspects of practising medicine when we get it right.

Box 7.1 Principles and tools to use when navigating dry rot

Principle	Gauge the patient's level of concern
Tools for assessing the patient's level of concern	*"How concerned are you about this?"* *"You seem quite worried about it"* *"Do you think it's serious?"*
Principle	Bridge any gap between your level of concern and the patient's by stating your own thoughts / concerns
Tools for explaining your thinking	*"The moles I take note of are the ones that look different to all the others"* *"I'm a bit worried that you have lost so much weight"* *"I do think we should take this seriously"*
Principle	Give space when breaking bad news
Tools for creating space	Use short sentences, with pauses and silence *"Your PSA test is very high,"* (pause) *"which does mean that this could be prostate cancer..."* (silence) *"There is a lot of sugar in your urine... I think the reason why you have not been feeling right is diabetes..."* (silence)
Principle	Don't be afraid to name it
Tools for naming the unmentionable	*"Of course, the thing we don't want to miss is bowel cancer"* *"This could be nothing, but because the blood is still present in your urine we should consider the possibility that it could be a cancer of the bladder"* *"Have you thought that this might be something like multiple sclerosis?"*

Chapter 8

Tending the garden

Make every contact count?

> **Shall we just get it over with?**
>
> I recognise the signs now. They vary, of course. Sometimes it is the slight drop of the shoulders, the hangdog expression, the look of learned helplessness and defeat. Or it might be just the opposite – the set jaw and steely look in the eye that say, *"Go on, then! Just you try, I'm ready for you!"*
>
> It usually happens in the second half of the consultation. We have talked about the problem, looked at the offending body part that has caused the symptoms and begun to skirt around the cause or hint at solutions, but we both know it is coming. There is no way around it – we are going to have to talk about weight. Maybe the best thing we can do is get it over with as quickly and as painlessly as possible.

I feel for my overweight patients. They can lie to me about how much they drink and admit to only half the cigarettes they smoke; they can even claim to actually get their money's worth from their gym subscription and I will happily believe them, but they cannot leave their weight at home when they visit me or pretend it isn't there. They know their heartburn / diabetes / foot pain / arthritis is partly due to their weight and all they can do is prepare themselves for a lecture.

It is bad enough that patients might feel told off when their lifestyle has contributed to their health problem, but the increasing emphasis on prevention and health promotion in recent years has led to initiatives such as *Make Every Contact Count*[1], where the expectation is to address lifestyle issues *every time* there is contact with a health professional. Patients might come about a cough, a cold or a wart on their finger and I am meant to talk to them about their weight. At their wits' end with depression, troubled by their periods, fed up with their psoriasis or worried about an elderly relative – if it looks like they might be on the heavy side then I am

---

1. NHS Future Forum (2012) *NHS Future Forum: summary report – second phase*. NHS.

to *make every contact count* and talk about weight reduction. And while we are at it, what about their smoking, drinking and that underused gym subscription...?

Not that a well-timed lecture can't have a dramatic effect. I well remember reviewing a patient in clinic one time who had made a good recovery from an episode of angina and he was keen that I passed on his thanks to the junior doctor who had first seen him. *"She saved my life, doctor"* he said. *"She told me I'd die if I didn't stop smoking. You know what I did? I handed over my packet of fags and haven't touched one since; best thing that could've happened to me!"*

I reassured him that I would certainly pass on his thanks to the doctor, and was glad for his success; what I did *not* tell him, however, was that my colleague had smoked every one of his cigarettes – *"shame to waste them,"* she had told me.

There is a fundamental difference between being in possession of medical knowledge and deciding to act on it

What this incident illustrates is the fundamental difference between being in possession of medical knowledge and deciding to act upon it – or, in the language of the cycle of change[2], moving from being pre-contemplative about change to actually taking action. My medical colleague undoubtedly knew more than most about the risks of smoking, yet she persisted despite the urgent advice she gave to her patient; the presence of crushing chest pain, however, was clearly capable of bringing the same advice into such sharp focus that it motivated radical change.

Primary care can undoubtedly play an important role in health promotion, and by encouraging a healthier lifestyle we may be the catalyst for significant health benefits. In reality, however, bringing about change is the exception and not the rule; more commonly, attempts to *make every contact count* are met with resistance, or even hostility. This is because, while it is entirely possible that our health advice could be in line with the patient's agenda, it is often significantly at odds with their purpose for making the appointment, or even contrary to their entire health belief system. What is more, health promotion is no longer just a matter of giving healthy lifestyle advice, but it has become medicalised due to increased understanding of the risk factors for disease, and the accompanying medical treatments that aim to modify these risk factors. These include medication for blood pressure, cholesterol, type 2 diabetes and osteoporosis, antithrombotic

2. Miller, W. R. and Rollnick, S. (1991) *Motivational Interviewing: preparing people to change addictive behavior.* Guilford Press.

treatments and all manner of health screening; this medicalisation of health has taken us from simple health promotion into the area of *chronic disease management*.

As with every aspect of the consultation, the challenge and the joy of the encounter is that we work with individuals rather than whole populations. While there may be an evidence base for encouraging a healthy lifestyle at a population level, we work with patients one at a time, each with their own unique set of health beliefs, idiosyncrasies and contradictions; and when it comes to health promotion and chronic disease management, those individual traits are more evident than ever.

Introducing the garden

Since both health promotion and chronic disease management do have an important place in the GP consultation, we need to consider how these apparent tasks fit into the *Two Houses* model. On the surface they are no different to any other problem we may be faced with: we may work out that *what matters* are issues related to health promotion or chronic disease management and we can decide what to do about this in the *House of Decision* in the same way as if the patient had presented with an acute problem. However, there is something here that *feels* very different to the core GP role of tending to the sick, so what is it that makes it distinct, and what does this mean for the consultation?

There are two key features that characterise this area of medicine:

1. One way or another, the initiative behind health promotion or chronic disease management has usually been led by the doctor, or at least by the medical profession as a whole (perhaps in the form of health awareness campaigns or invitation to screening programmes, for instance), and not by the patient's symptoms.
2. The problems being addressed are not one-off problems to be dealt with and left behind, but need ongoing maintenance and monitoring.

Within the *Two Houses* model I have chosen to imagine this part of the consultation taking place in the *garden* rather than within the walls of one of the houses, since it helps us to keep these two key features in mind.

The garden as a separate space

Since the garden is separate from the house this reminds us that there may be tension between the need to attend to chronic disease management and any acute problem the patient may have come with. This tension can work both ways. The patient may come about a distinct problem, such as a painful knee, while the doctor is bombarded with pop-up alerts advising that there are overdue checks to attend to; we can imagine the doctor feeling pressure to pull the patient out of the house and into the garden in order to do this. Or the patient may have come for their medication review, but wants to talk about their knee while they have the doctor's time; here the consultation starts in the garden, but the patient expects the doctor to simultaneously attend to a need in the house.

By thinking of chronic disease management as separate in this way we can anticipate the problems that arise when the priorities of the doctor and patient are different. We should not be surprised when the patient becomes frustrated if the doctor seems to be preoccupied with their blood pressure when they have come to talk about their knee, or that it is stressful for the doctor to conduct a medication review and be presented with a list of acute problems at the same time! The doctor and patient can easily become embroiled in a tug of war between the house and the garden; the doctor needs to develop the skills to avoid this conflict and find a way to walk with the patient seamlessly between the two.

The doctor and patient can easily become embroiled in a tug of war between the house and the garden

The garden as a space that requires maintenance

The imagery of a garden also naturally lends itself to recognising the importance of regular maintenance. Just as a garden will become untidy and wild if left unattended, so chronic disease management will slip over time. Successful lifestyle changes may lapse, blood pressure may rise and diabetes checks need to be done. We can imagine such maintenance in the consulting room as the equivalent of regular weeding and pruning, with different areas of the garden needing attention depending on the underlying problem, whether it be a medical 'chronic disease' such as hypertension or osteoporosis, or a lifestyle factor such as exercise or smoking.

While neglecting a garden for too long can lead to greater problems down the line, gardening is rarely so urgent that it must be done today. There are days when it is raining too heavily to even go outside and others where the conditions are perfect and we make real headway against the ever-present weeds. So too with health promotion and chronic disease management. We should not keep kicking the can down the road, but there are consultations where there is the equivalent of heavy rain: when more urgent clinical need takes priority or someone has just been bereaved, for instance; or maybe the patient list is just too long and the best we can manage is to get the ball rolling with setting routine blood tests in place, or arranging some home blood pressure monitoring and a plan to meet again.

Gardening as a useful shorthand

You may have noticed by now that 'health promotion and chronic disease management' is something of a mouthful; I have certainly been aware of how often I have typed that phrase so far in this chapter, but I cannot think of a simpler medical term that covers all aspects of this side of medicine. To consider this part of the consultation as 'gardening' may be helpful here. During the consultation we can ask ourselves questions like: 'Do we need to do any gardening?'; 'Is this the right time and place to garden?'; 'Is this a new opportunity to tackle something in the garden?' When teaching the consultation we can ask our trainees to think in this way, and when covering clinical topics we can encourage them to include a section on the garden, so that it becomes second nature for them to consider what might happen in this particular space.

Manicured lawn or untamed wilderness?

For those of us lucky enough to have an outside space, the garden is one area of our home that is frequently either the most loved or the most neglected. Some of us will have beautifully tended lawns, deep flowerbeds teeming with colourful herbaceous perennials, or cultivated raised beds bursting with fruit and vegetables. Others will enjoy a more carefree approach to gardening, where weeds and flowers compete in some sort of ordered chaos, the lawn is mown only when it gets too long to play football and the only produce is an ancient apple tree that supplies more shade than apples. For many, however, the garden will be a wilderness, so overgrown with brambles and stinging nettles that any attempt to control it is quickly reversed and where the owners have long since given up the garden as a usable space and learnt to hide away from it.

When it comes to health promotion and chronic disease management there are many similarities with these different approaches to gardening. Some of our patients will be keen to have regular health checks and attend reliably for their reviews, complete with a beautiful Excel spreadsheet of home blood pressure readings, occasionally even with detailed statistical analysis. Others will take note of some health advice, but ignore most of it, attend for reviews with a bit of prompting and consider some medication to reduce future risk, but only go so far. Still others will only darken our door when their symptoms are troublesome enough that they have no option and resist all attempts for the consultation to deviate from addressing the presenting problem.

When we delve into the realm of health promotion and disease prevention, therefore, we can consider ourselves to be asking the patient to allow us to venture into the very personal space of their garden, with all of its idiosyncrasies. If our time there is to prove fruitful then, before we start hacking back the shrubs or pulling out what we believe to be weeds, we must first attempt to understand the patient's own relationship with this complex area of their life. If we try to change someone's health-related behaviour we must expect to encounter strong feelings, such as pride, embarrassment, frustration, suspicion, fears, habitual behaviours and all sorts of ingrained health beliefs. When we learn to recognise these feelings and beliefs, and to respect them as much as we respect our own advice and the guidelines we follow, then we can start to become truly proficient gardeners.

Remember who owns the garden

The medical profession has language it uses for when patients don't go along with our advice. 'Non-compliance' is one of the most common terms for when patients do not take their medication as prescribed. The dictionary definition for non-compliance is 'a failure to act in accordance with a wish or command' while the word compliance implies passivity on the part of the patient, and that they should bend to the doctor's will. Is such a paternalistic term really how we want to describe what is happening here?

Disobedience

I was chatting to a good friend recently. *"I'm starting to rattle,"* he told me. *"My doctor's put me on blood pressure tablets now."*

In fact, he was now on two tablets, so hardly rattling compared to some of my patients, but he is in good health and only in his fifties, so I could see where he was coming from. It turned out he had undertaken 24-hour blood pressure monitoring.

"I took it off half the time," he told me. *"I just couldn't sleep with it on, and it was such a pain when you're driving as you never know when it's going to go off."* I nodded and sighed, thinking of how many patients have told me the same thing and yet the medical establishment continues to consider it as the gold standard.

And what of the result? *"132 over 86,"* he told me. *"She said that they like it to be 85 or lower so I should take a tablet. I didn't think it was that different, but she seemed pretty keen I started something."*

I didn't know quite what to say. My sympathies lay with my friend, but I could also imagine a GP looking at the hypertension guidelines and worrying about doing the wrong thing if she didn't recommend treatment. What intrigued me was what my friend said next.

"So I'm breaking them in half and just taking half a tablet. I haven't told her as I don't want to seem ungrateful, but I think it will be OK."

It is a term that has been questioned in recent years, and 'non-concordance' has been suggested as an alternative. This is certainly better, but even non-concordance means non-agreement and we should ask where the problem lies when this happens; is such non-agreement the fault of the patient, or a failure to achieve a shared understanding where the patient's only course of action is to reject a plan they did not feel sufficiently part of?

Nor is this the only example of such doctor-centred language. The Quality and Outcomes Framework is a key part of the GP contract in the UK and sets targets for GPs in an attempt to improve care and monitoring of chronic disease such as hypertension, diabetes and so on. Since there is an understanding

The enforced use of the language of disobedience and rebellion is entirely inappropriate

that not all patients can be expected to achieve strict targets, the GP is allowed to exempt some patients from the calculations on the grounds of extra treatment being inappropriate, or on the basis of patient choice.

However, I am not permitted to describe this as the patient's choice, but have to label such a decision as 'informed dissent'. This enforced use of the language of disobedience and rebellion whenever a patient declines the suggestion of extra treatment is entirely inappropriate; because the patient is free to make their own choices in their garden, how can they be disobedient? That would mean rebelling against themselves!

When it comes to disease prevention it is essential that doctors remember at all times who the garden belongs to, and that it is the patient who should decide what they would like to happen in their garden. The doctor is the visitor to this place and, while we have been invited in as a professional to help, advise and encourage good gardening, we must always remember that it is not the doctor who has the ultimate authority here.

Correct use of guidelines

Guidelines have become central to the practice of modern medicine, and are extremely important, but it is helpful to remember that they are mostly there as a reminder of best practice, and to curtail maverick doctors, not maverick patients. A guideline on the treatment of a urinary tract infection, for instance, will help me know when to consider using antibiotics, and give guidance on which antibiotics to use, thus preventing me from going straight to some broad-spectrum antibiotic which works well, but will contribute to resistance problems. I am not allowed to be a maverick and prescribe whatever I want. When it comes to whether or not the patient actually wishes to take an antibiotic, this is usually dictated by the degree to which they are bothered by their symptoms; how, then, should we approach guidelines when this pressure to treat is absent, because there *are* no symptoms? Guidelines on the prevention of disease, such as hypertension or osteoporosis, or on the use of statins generally fall into this category, and it is essential that the doctor recognises this fundamental difference when it comes to their application.

Guidelines are there to curtail maverick doctors, not maverick patients

Ben Goldacre and Liam Smeeth wrote a fascinating *BMJ* editorial on this subject in 2014, arguing that when we offer preventive drugs to healthy people,

> *"... we are a long way from the doctor treating a sick patient. In some respects, we are less like doctors and more like a*

life insurance sales team: offering occasional, possibly life changing, benefits, many years from now, in exchange for small ongoing inconvenience and cost."[3]

This is a hugely important insight. We know that taking a tablet like a statin will have a significant benefit for some people, but make no difference to the outcome for the majority, since in only a small number of those who take it will it prevent an event that would have happened if they had not taken it. Unlike insurance, however, when each person subscribing to the insurance will know whether or not they have made a claim, there is the complication that those who have benefited from medication for disease prevention have no way of knowing that they have prevented a future event. We should not be surprised, therefore, if different patients have very different views on taking out such 'insurance', or if their views are much more diverse than whether or not they want to take antibiotics for a painful urine infection.

What should we make of guidelines, for instance, that recommend a statin to anyone with a ten-year cardiovascular disease risk of greater than 10%? The key word in such guidelines is that such treatment should be *offered*. That is to say that we have permission to prescribe statins in these circumstances, and some obligation to discuss it with the patient. Again, this prevents the maverick doctor from prescribing statins outside of such guidance, but it does leave plenty of room for patient choice. How do they feel about taking a tablet every day? What is their approach to risk? How much time and energy are they willing to dedicate towards disease prevention? Are they ready to change their lifestyle? With the absence of symptoms to drive treatment, the answers to these questions become the centre ground of achieving a shared understanding and so a shared management plan.

The garden as a dynamic space

Since our attitude to risk management dramatically influences how we tend our garden, and how we want the doctor to help us tend it, it is well worth investing time to discover what our patients really think and feel about their garden – because to truly understand the patient's relationship with their garden will not only help the consultation we are in the middle

3. Goldacre, B. and Smeeth, L. (2014) Mass treatment with statins. *BMJ*, **349:** g4745.

of today, but consultations for years to come. These attitudes are not fixed, however, but may change in time. A young man might start to pay more attention to his lifestyle once he becomes a father, for instance, or crosses the milestone of a significant birthday; a woman might be influenced by seeing her ageing mother hunched over as the result of osteoporotic fractures. Such events are cues for the doctor to look out for, and to use tactfully to help bring about behavioural change.

What is more, the actions we take when tending the garden – such as starting treatment for blood pressure or helping achieve behavioural change – will affect the nature of this space in the patient's life from that time on. The patient may now have become an ex-smoker and the garden feels a better place for them to enjoy, or they may have been started on treatment for cholesterol and, while we may be helpfully preventing disease, their garden is forever changed by such an act. They will be reminded of this change, for better or for worse, every evening when they take their tablet. They will need to remember to order repeat prescriptions and put aside time for reviews and blood tests. Many patients will welcome such intervention; perhaps the nightly routine will be a comforting reminder that they are doing what they can to reduce the chance of having a stroke like their father, for instance. On the other hand, they may be burdened by it as they somehow feel they have been medicalised and their previously private garden has an unwelcome intruder. What the doctor must do is be mindful of the impact of our recommendations and treatments on the individual in front of us. When it comes to disease prevention, the words of Susan Sontag are worth keeping in mind whenever we find ourselves recommending treatment. Written over 40 years ago, they are perhaps even more relevant now than they were in 1978:

> *"Illness is the night-side of life, a more onerous citizenship. Everyone who is born holds dual citizenship, in the kingdom of the well and in the kingdom of the sick. Although we all prefer to use only the good passport, sooner or later each of us is obliged, at least for a spell, to identify ourselves as citizens of that other place."*[4]

The issue with modern medicine is that, more often than not, it is not illness that makes us identify with *"that other place"*, but disease prevention; we should not be surprised that some patients are reluctant citizens.

---

4. Sontag, S. (1978) *Illness as Metaphor*. Farrar, Straus and Giroux.

Further reading – motivational interviewing and gift-wrapping

When we enter the garden we frequently encounter the challenge of enabling behavioural change, a task full of hazardous pitfalls and with the potential to cause endless frustration, since human beings rarely do what they are told! How to motivate people to change their behaviour is complex and far beyond the remit of this book, but healthcare professionals will find their work is much more rewarding if they can familiarise themselves with some of the excellent work in this area. Here I would point the reader to the work of Miller and Rollnick[5] on the principles of motivational interviewing, a clinical method developed for use in psychology, but much of which can be applied to general practice, even within the confines of a ten-minute consultation.

And finally, it is well worth remembering Neighbour's description of gift-wrapping, described in *The Inner Consultation*[6]. This concept is less well known than his ideas of summarising and safety-netting but is an incredibly important principle to keep in mind when negotiating a plan. Neighbour reminds us that when we share a proposed plan with a patient it always comes 'gift-wrapped' in the language we choose to use, the pace of delivery and so on. We should aim to make this metaphorical wrapping paper as helpful as possible to the individual patient we are working with, so that they can relate to it and find it acceptable – for example, by using our prior knowledge of the patient and incorporating the patient's own language and health beliefs as the shared plan is developed.

5. Miller, W.R. and Rollnick, S. (1991) *Motivational Interviewing: preparing people to change addictive behavior.* Guilford Press.

6. Neighbour, R. (2015) *The Inner Consultation*, 2nd edition. CRC Press.

Box 8.1 Principles and tools to apply to tending the garden

Principle: discover what the patient thinks before recommending change	Find out if the patient is ready to consider a lifestyle change
Tools to discover the patient's views in a non-judgemental way	*"What are your thoughts on smoking?"* *"How do you feel about your weight?"* *"I'm a bit worried about your drinking"*
Principle: check with the patient before you move into the garden	Make sure that the patient is ready to move with you when you move between the house and garden
Tools for keeping the patient with you	*"We can certainly look at your knee while you are here; would it be OK if we checked your blood pressure first?"* *"We do need to do your medication review, but the problem with your bowels also sounds important; which would you like us to focus on today?"* *"As we've decided to concentrate on your headaches today, how about I give you something to read about cholesterol and we talk about that properly next time?"*
Principle: understand the patient's priorities	Help the patient weigh up the costs and benefits of disease prevention
Tools to help the patient express their views	*"What are your thoughts on statins?"* *"You mentioned that your husband is on a statin, how does he find it?"* *"How important is it to you to try to prevent something like a stroke?"* *"How do you feel about taking a tablet every day?"*
Principle: understand behavioural change	Utilise the principles of motivational interviewing
Tools to explore ambivalence in behavioural change	*"I know you would prefer to not take tablets, but your high blood pressure is also worrying you – how do we square that one?"* *"So, you would like to stop smoking, but you're not sure you can right now; how will you know when the time is right to stop?"*

Principle: make the plan personalised	Gift-wrap the plan in a way that is acceptable to the patient
Tools to use for gift-wrapping a plan	*"I could prescribe peppermint oil capsules, or if you want to keep it simple, you could try peppermint tea first"*
	"I wonder if we could avoid using tablets at all if we could really work on the lifestyle side of this"
	"You've always said to me that you don't want to end up with a crumpled spine like your mother; maybe we should consider treatment to protect your bones"

Chapter 9

A house with two wings

The *House of Decision*

This is the most important chapter in this book.

It concerns the point of transition where the consultation moves from the *House of Discovery* to the *House of Decision*; a key moment where doctor and patient can move smoothly in tandem to a shared management plan, or become damagingly disengaged, derailing a consultation that appeared to be going well until this point. There is a natural change of tempo between the two houses, with the emphasis shifting from listening and inquiry towards decision and action. This increased dynamism is often more comfortable for the doctor than the patient, and plays into the medical inclination to try to fix everything. As a result, a startling amnesia can develop in the doctor's consciousness, so that they fail to act on what the patient has said up until this point and their thinking becomes overly coloured by their own viewpoint, concerns about following guidelines, or both.

> **A startling amnesia can develop in the doctor's consciousness**

There is no doubt that the second half of the consultation is more difficult to get right than its predecessor. Partly this is because it can only build on the foundations of what has gone before, so that a poor first half usually leads to an equally dysfunctional ending. Moreover, the second half takes longer to perfect because we get to practise it less.

Music lessons

When my daughter was young and learning to play the piano, she would always start practising her pieces from the beginning. As a result, the first page would be mastered well before the end of the piece; many times I would listen to her, thinking she had cracked it until she turned the page and her fingers would start to trip over the less familiar passages in the second half. There was a feedback loop that enforced this phenomenon, since becoming accomplished with the beginning of a piece increased the enjoyment of playing it, and so the inclination to practise it, while the last page would be visited only begrudgingly and always seemed more difficult. I have often thought the same is true of GP registrars as they set out in primary care. As they practise the consultation so the beginning increases in familiarity, and the skills required, such as learning to listen or establish rapport, become well established. As each consultation progresses, however, many will go off-piste; the registrar may have to ask their trainer who ends up taking over, or they lose structure and are never quite sure where it went wrong, or the patient accepts the plan, but they didn't quite connect. The end result is fewer opportunities to practise and master the second half, compounded by the fact that there are so many directions that this part of the consultation can head in that it is impossible to practise them all. The end result is that the *House of Decision* becomes so much more difficult to master than the *House of Discovery*, and for this reason, rather like the last page in my daughter's piano pieces, it needs more attention to get it right.

A shared understanding

What is key to ensuring a smooth transition between the houses, and therefore a good outcome to the consultation, is the establishment of a *shared understanding*. The term that will be more familiar to doctors is *shared decision-making* (SDM), since there has been a welcome recognition within medicine in recent years of the importance of SDM in good clinical care. There are NICE guidelines on SDM, numerous SDM decision aids to share with patients, international conferences on the subject and even an International SDM Society.

Shared understanding requires the doctor to risk the implications of an equal meeting of minds

Anything that helps patients to be more involved in decisions about their health has to be a good thing, but it is a shame that the favoured term has become SDM, rather than *shared understanding*. SDM implies welcoming the patient into the doctor's world; the emphasis is most often placed on helping the patient to understand the technical complexities of each medical decision so that they can make an informed choice. This can become quite daunting, and well-intentioned decision aids that are meant to empower the patient can be simply overwhelming – for instance, the NICE Patient Decision Aid designed to help women decide whether or not to take medication to reduce the risk of breast cancer runs to nineteen pages of complex text, boxes and diagrams! Moreover, SDM narrows down the definition of what is shared to the area of decisions, with no commitment to a deeper shared experience between patient and doctor. *Shared understanding*, on the other hand, is a much broader and more balanced concept; it requires the doctor to recognise the patient's perspective, to venture into their world and to risk the implications of a much more equal meeting of minds. The patient, as the expert on themselves, their story, what matters to them and how their body feels, comes to a mutual understanding with the doctor, who puts their expertise at the patient's disposal to help guide them in the light of whatever problem they have brought to the consultation.

Richard Lehman, a GP whose insights, wit and wisdom were enjoyed by the profession for many years in his regular *BMJ* column, described *shared understanding* as *"the central challenge of medicine in this century"*[1]. In fact, he felt so strongly about it that he become the Professor of the Shared Understanding of Medicine at the University of Birmingham. I can't think of anyone better for the role, and I certainly share his passion for the challenge. Having said that, we can't possibly understand everything about the patient in the context of a brief consultation and so it is worth thinking about how we break this down – this is where the two wings come in.

A house with two wings

Hot under the collar

A friend of mine recently told me about an encounter she had had with her GP:

Several years ago, I saw a GP as I was having trouble sleeping. My heart felt as if it was trying to get out of my chest and I felt continuously sick and bloated. After ordering some blood tests and an ECG, she informed me that my hormone levels were low, indicating I was probably menopausal, and this was why I was feeling so awful. She then said she would prescribe sertraline as this had been known to help with hot flushes. I said there'd been a couple of times when I'd felt hot but I didn't really suffer from hot flushes. She still went ahead and gave me the prescription. I didn't feel as if I could argue, she seemed to be in a hurry and so I left.

1. Lehman, R. (2017) Richard Lehman's journal review. *The BMJ Opinion.* Available at: bit.ly/31qMMBN (accessed February 2020)

I went home with the sertraline and read the leaflet. I found that among its very common side-effects were sleep disorders, palpitations and nausea, as well as many other things. I had suffered from palpitations in the past (probably due to caffeine) and I knew my heart did the 'skippy' thing (is that arrhythmia?), and I already had nausea. I didn't feel safe taking this drug.

I went back to the GP and let her know my concerns about sertraline. She looked confused and said it was shown to be helpful with hot flushes. I said I didn't get hot flushes. She still looked confused. I told her I wasn't comfortable with strong drugs as I had a low threshold to everything. I told her I was trying over-the-counter things like Kalms to help me sleep and was having some success. She said that was fine but still recommended the sertraline.

I came away feeling like a 'bad patient'. I wasn't following doctor's orders to help me get well. If I didn't do as suggested or take what was offered, how could I expect to feel better? If she had acknowledged my anxieties and addressed them, or even said to try to continue without drugs, I would have felt better. All I really wanted to know was, was I dying? Was this normal for menopausal patients? Would this go away eventually? I accept that she was trying to relieve my symptoms but she just didn't understand that I may have something to say about my own treatment.

The doctor wanted to solve the problem, while the patient wanted a greater understanding of her situation

The problem with this consultation was that there was a mismatch between my friend and her doctor with regard to the desired outcome; the doctor wanted to solve the problem while my friend's main aim was to gain a greater understanding of her situation. In fact, the outcome of almost every consultation can be considered as a balance between these two key objectives:

1. For the patient to gain an *increased understanding* of their problem.
2. For the patient and doctor to work towards a *solution* to the problem.

These objectives are so fundamental that the *House of Decision* can be considered as having two wings – the *Increased Understanding* wing and the *Solutions* wing. We can then imagine that my friend was in one wing of the house, while the doctor was in the other, and the best they could do was to shout across the divide. Of course, it could happen just as well the other way around. We have all been there when we think we have done a good job reassuring someone that their chest pain is not from their heart and that they don't need to worry about it when, at the last minute, the patient says, *"So what are you going to do about my pain, doctor?"* We have spent all our time in the *Increased Understanding* wing of the house and missed the fact that they also wanted us to *do* something about their pain – in other words, they also wanted to visit the *Solutions* wing. In reality, most patients will want to spend some time in both wings and the best consultations occur when the doctor and patient are able to gain a truly shared understanding of the relative priorities of these two destinations.

Looking for cues

Most of the groundwork for determining which wing should take priority, or whether both are equally important, is performed through careful listening while in the *House of Discovery*. Sometimes the patient will overtly signal their intended destination in the second house with statements like, *"I was wondering if I might need physiotherapy"* or *"I just want to make sure it's nothing to worry about"* but frequently the cues are more subtle. Statements like:

"I can't live like this"

"This is the third time I've come back"

and *"I don't want another night like that"*

all imply that the patient is looking for a solution to their problem, while:

"I'm just a bit worried about it"

"I don't want to waste your time, but..."

or *"I'm just not sure what it is"*

might suggest that the patient is more interested in an explanation for their symptoms than the need to find a solution. Like all cues, however, these are hints to what the patient is thinking rather than clear statements and will need to be explored further. Asking directly what the patient is looking for can be very helpful here, with questions such as:

"Is it more important for you to understand what is happening here, or to find a way to get rid of these symptoms?"

"So if we were confident that your pain wasn't being caused by anything serious, how would you feel about the pain then?"

"It sounds like you are keen to do something about this, is that right?"

Of course, this all comes under the heading of exploring the patient's expectations, as described by Pendleton, but at this very fundamental level of seeking either understanding, a solution, or both, it is much easier for the patient to contribute. We are not asking them to come up with a formulated plan, so much as checking the general direction of travel. Most patients will be able to give very helpful answers to such questions, compared with the much lower rate of return with a more demanding 'expectation' question such as, *"So did you have any thoughts of what we might do next?"* which, as discussed in the first chapter, often elicits the reply, *"No, not really"*. It may seem odd to consider the 'yield' a doctor gets from asking certain questions, but just as we learn the usefulness of tests we order, or the examination techniques we use, so too we gain a feel for the yield of the questions we ask. Questions with a low yield will soon be discarded, no matter how noble their intent. Starting to find out the patient's expectations at the level of wanting greater understanding or a working towards a solution will bring much more satisfying results, encouraging the doctor to ask them more often, and refine them so that such an approach becomes an unconscious skill.

A crucial factor in achieving *shared understanding* is to discover the patient's prior understanding of their problem, but just as important is to place their prior knowledge within their own narrative. Three patients might have an identical understanding of the technical aspects of depression, for instance, but one has parents who have always been very judgemental about anything to do with mental health; another has a highly supportive partner, but he doesn't want to burden her as she is going through treatment for breast cancer; while the third is worried about what this will mean for her ambition to join the army. The doctor cannot understand what the illness journey will be like for these patients without creating an environment where these stories can be shared and listened to. Indeed, it may be that the majority of the shared understanding is from the patient to the doctor, and that just voicing their story and being heard reflects back a greater level of understanding in itself, with the doctor acting primarily as a catalyst.

However, there is usually also a need for the doctor to share their own understanding; after all, when asked what they think is going on, many patients rightly say, *"If I knew that, I wouldn't be here!"* – they want and expect to know what the doctor thinks. There will be examination findings to describe, symptoms to try to explain and possible diagnoses to consider. Some of this will involve the doctor simply explaining their thinking, which is one of the most powerful tools in the consultation. Examples of how such explanations could take shape include:

> *"I'm just wondering if these could be migraines"*

> *"Well, the things we need to consider when you have pain just below the ribs like this are problems with stomach acid, or perhaps gallstones"*

> *"Diarrhoea can often last up to a week when we have a tummy bug, but when it lasts much longer than that I tend to think it needs looking into"*

What is important in statements like this is that they can be used before the doctor has drawn firm conclusions; they are pointers to what the doctor is thinking, but leave room for the patient to contribute and can be open to redirection. The more the doctor values the patient's role, the more effective this will be. The questions above, for instance, might elicit the following replies:

> *"They're not like my usual migraines"*

> *"Yes, I was wondering if it might be an ulcer"*

> *"I'm glad you said that, it doesn't seem right that it's gone on this long"*

each of which would have a significant impact on the direction of the consultation. Of course, if the patient challenges a hypothesis that does not mean they are right, but the fact that they have challenged it will always be significant. With the migraines, for instance, the doctor may respond to the patient's comment by rejecting this diagnosis, but if the doctor still has good reason to think they are migraines it is important to consider why the patient thinks they are not. What are the 'usual migraines' like? How do these headaches

Statements about what the doctor is thinking can be used before the doctor has drawn firm conclusions, leaving room for the patient to contribute

differ? Are they worried that there is something more serious going on than migraines? If the doctor can understand this context then a shared understanding of the current headaches is much more likely.

Formulating understanding 'on the go' like this can be unsettling, especially for trainees for whom the hospital model discourages such an approach. With a hospital clerking, the doctor records all aspects of the history and examination, then usually takes this away to consider in the light of any investigations, or after a discussion with seniors, before returning to the patient to explain the diagnosis and management plan. While this can work in a secondary care setting, it encourages trainees to think that they should have a fully formulated diagnosis and management plan before they share it with the patient. Sharing their thinking before this process is completed might be seen as a sign of weakness, or even being unprofessional. In reality, sharing thinking like this, when done well, increases the sense of shared working with the patient, brings their experience and perspective to the problem and helps ensure better decisions. Trainees often find that the difficult decisions they are faced with become much easier to manage once they learn to trust the patient in this way.

Once a clear idea of the nature of the problem has been established, there may be a need to share technical medical understanding with the patient, and we might consider that one of the most significant rooms in the *Increased Understanding* wing of the *House of Decision* is the High Tech Room – the complexities of which will be discussed in the next chapter.

A network of rooms

Both wings in the *House of Decision* can be considered as a network of rooms, some in parallel along a corridor, others leading off one another or interconnected in some other way. Aside from the High Tech Room (see *Chapter 10*), each room contains some action or decision. This is a dynamic, changeable house whose rooms vary depending on the problem; for a shoulder problem, for instance, the main rooms would include physiotherapy, painkillers, a steroid injection or referral to consider a scan or surgery; when the problem is hypertension there could be rooms containing antihypertensives, weight loss, salt reduction or other lifestyle measures, as well as further investigations that could be arranged. There is no limit to the number of rooms, and when the doctor and patient work well together they may find rooms that neither had expected; for instance, the patient might like to just monitor their blood pressure for the moment as they are about to retire and hope this will improve things, or they might decide that t'ai chi would be a gentler option for their shoulder pain. The objective of some of these rooms is to gain information; for instance rooms that include arranging investigations, watchful waiting or a trial of treatment. Such rooms might be considered to be located in the *Increased Understanding* wing, while others, which may contain medication, an operation or therapy, are best thought of as being in the *Solutions* wing.

The challenge for the doctor is how to approach these rooms. Atul Gawande, in his truly excellent book *Being Mortal*[2], describes two approaches doctors frequently take, both of which are problematic.

1. **The paternalistic approach**

    Here, the doctor chooses to give direct advice to the patient about the best course of action – the equivalent of taking the patient by the hand to the doctor's preferred room, opening the door and telling them that this is the best solution for them. While this might be appropriate when there really is only one sensible option, thankfully this doctor-centred approach has increasingly been rejected by patients and doctors alike. There is a risk, however, that the rising dominance of guidelines in clinical practice could reverse this trend, as the fear of operating outside guidelines threatens to become the new controlling voice in the consulting room, encouraging guideline-centred paternalism.

2. **Informative approach**

    Here the patient is given all the information they need to make their own decision and is asked to choose – the equivalent of throwing open all the doors in the *House of Decision* and saying *"There you go, which do you want?"* This approach may be more patient-centred, but it still causes problems, since the patient can be left floundering, unsure of which way to turn as the doctor has abdicated any sense of leadership.

A friend of mine said to me recently, *"I know you're not allowed to tell us what to do these days, but I wish you doctors would give us some guidance sometimes!"* She has a good point, and it is fascinating that the profession has left her feeling like this so often that she has concluded we are *not allowed* to guide her any more! As Gawande says, the purely informative approach is more like being a retail sales person than a doctor – and a poor retailer at that.

---

2. Gawande, A. (2015) *Being Mortal: illness, medicine, and what matters in the end*. Profile Books.

I remember a much more positive retail experience when I went with my daughter to buy an electric piano. The shop was bewildering, with dozens of keyboards on display and a great deal of technical information to take on board, but I remember clearly the helpful approach of the shop assistant. He did three things: he gave us time, shared his expertise when we needed him to, and listened to our priorities so that he could help us to achieve our goals. We were never left floundering with too much choice, nor did he railroad us into making a decision, but neither did we need to obtain anything like his level of understanding in order to make the right choice.

Sharing options should involve listening to the priorities of the patient and then using our expertise to help bring the plan into line with these priorities. For instance, when it comes to treating high cholesterol with a statin, how does the patient balance their feeling about being on a tablet all the time against the risk of stroke if they don't? How does the doctor's analysis of their individual stroke risk influence this balance? If a patient has a knee problem, how much are they prepared to go through to get it sorted? Would they consider surgery, or are they not ready for that yet? We can consider that each room in the *Solutions* wing contains both a reward (the potential that it might improve the problem) and a cost (potential for side-effects, pain or stress involved in treatment, investment of time, changes to the patient's perception of themselves, etc.). For each room, the patient will be balancing the reward against the cost, both of which will be different for every patient, as they make their decisions. The doctor needs to explore these rewards and costs, so that the patient is not left on their own in the decision-making process, but, through shared understanding, is offered guidance and leadership by an informed doctor, helping them to navigate the rooms in the *House of Decision* together.

> **Sharing options should involve listening to the priorities of the patient and then using our expertise to help bring the plan into line with these**

While the contents in the rooms of this house will vary depending on the nature of the problem, there are certain types of room to look out for which will come up time and again, each with its own challenges and opportunities; these include Empty Rooms, Locked Rooms, Hidden Rooms, Optional rooms and Room 101. Each will be considered in detail in *Chapters 11, 12* and *13*, but first we will navigate the High Tech Room in *Chapter 10*.

Box 9.1 Principles and tools to apply to achieve shared understanding

Principle: watch out for cues	Always consider the balance between the need for *increased understanding* and finding a *solution*
Tools for listening to cues	Cues that imply a need for *increased understanding:* **"I just don't know what's going on"** **"It's worrying me now"** **"My family told me to come"** Cues that imply a need to work towards a *solution:* **"I don't want to get fobbed off again"** **"I've got to get back to work"** **"This can't go on"**
Principle: clarify your shared understanding	It can be helpful to explore the patient's desired outcome in terms of *increased understanding* and working towards a *solution*
Tools for clarifying the desired outcome	*"How keen are you to find a solution for this problem?"* *"Were you looking to understand what's going on, or are you more interested in finding a solution?"* *"Are you at the point where you would like to get something done about this?"* *"If we were sure this was nothing serious, how would you feel about living with these symptoms?"*
Principle: don't be afraid to mould the plan with the patient	Explain your thinking 'on the go' so that the patient is included and can contribute along the way – adapt your thinking according to what they say
Tools to use to explain your thinking	*"A key thing we need to think about here is whether to go up to the hospital or manage this at home"* *"I'm wondering if your body is trying to tell you that it needs a rest"* *"We obviously don't want to miss a serious cause for your headache, but it could be something quite simple like pressure in your sinuses"*

Chapter 10

The High Tech Room

When our dishwasher packed up a few years ago, I described the symptoms to the engineer as he arrived and watched as he performed his examination; now he was ready to deliver his verdict. In the language of the *Two Houses* model, we had left the *House of Discovery* and were about to enter the *House of Decision*. I was interested in visiting both wings of this house. I was mostly seeking a solution so that I could wash the dishes, but I also wanted to understand the problem – and for that we had to visit the High Tech Room. The engineer called me over to the broken dishwasher, holding a gadget in his hand that was some kind of probe with a digital display. He thrust the device into the bowels of the machine, sucked air through his teeth and shook his head.

"That's 8.5, that is," he said, showing me the digital display.

To this day I don't know what the device was or what 8.5 meant, other than that he deemed it to be terminal. I don't know if it was too high or too low, what might have caused it or how to prevent such a calamity in a future machine. I could have asked for more details, of course, but he made no attempt to enlighten me, and by this point I had so little confidence in him that I just wanted him to leave. As an attempt to try to avoid replacing the dishwasher, it proved a complete waste of time and money, but as an object lesson in what it feels like to be on the receiving end of the High Tech Room, I'm sure it will stay with me longer than our new dishwasher.

We all have times when we are obliged to enter an unfamiliar technical arena – taking the car to the garage or the daunting prospect of needing an accountant for the first time at the end of GP training are obvious examples – and it is useful to keep in mind what this feels like, since most of our patients are in this position every time we see them. If it is stressful trying to understand the implications of a faulty dishwasher or a worn-out camshaft, when ultimately we are only talking about a piece of machinery, then how much more difficult must it be to navigate medical problems when it could be our very lives at stake?

The High Tech Room is not a cosy consultation room, replete with comfy sofas, but is instead inescapably technical. We can imagine it like entering an air traffic control room, packed with complex visual displays, arrays of numbers and machines that go 'beep'. Our world is full of medical terminology to navigate, numbers to explain and test results to interpret:

The High Tech Room is not a cosy consultation room, replete with comfy sofas

what does 'mild left ventricular impairment' actually mean for the patient? Why have you said I have 'chronic kidney *disease*'? Is a cholesterol of 5.5 something I have to worry about? The list is endless, and the challenge for the doctor is how to explain our world in a way that is meaningful and relevant without overwhelming the patient or patronising them in the process. It is one of the hardest tasks we have to do.

Mrs Jones comes for her blood results

When we taught information-giving on the Guildford training scheme we always acted out a sketch for the trainees where poor Mrs Jones (or Mr Jones, depending on who was in which role that day) came to see the doctor for her blood results. Her HbA1c was raised at 85 mmol/mol and this was the first time she would be told that she has diabetes.

The doctor always started the scenario with a pile of boxes of all sorts of shapes and sizes next to their chair and would take the largest of these as Mrs Jones entered the room, passing it over to her at the moment they gave the diagnosis of diabetes. From this point on, the doctor would keep picking up boxes, and would hand one over with each new piece of information:

- Diabetes meant her blood sugars were too high – a shoebox
- High sugars could cause her arteries to fur up – an unmarked black box
- Her blood pressure was up so she should do some home monitoring – an eggbox
- Her feet need to be checked – a shoebox; and her kidneys – another eggbox
- There are dietary changes she needs to make – a chocolate box
- She should cut down on alcohol – a wine box
- She would be referred to get the back of her eyes photographed – a glasses case
- She'll get an appointment with the dietitian – a sweet box

Mrs Jones would do her best to add each box to the mounting pile on her lap, gradually disappearing from the doctor's view as the boxes accumulated. More boxes would be added – an appointment in the diabetic clinic; advice about cholesterol; referral to an educational programme; starting treatment with metformin. The last box was always the smallest and was given with a closing flourish as she was asked to bring a urine sample to her next appointment.

Overwhelmed and despondent, Mrs Jones would stand up, trying in vain to juggle the mountain of boxes on her lap and the doctor would take no notice of the boxes spilling all over the floor as she left.

When we asked the trainees for feedback at the end of the course, the image of Mrs Jones dropping her boxes was often one of the more memorable images they were left with, and it is worth remembering whenever we find ourselves with a lot of information we want to impart. It is well known that patients retain a disappointing proportion of what we say to them, but to imagine them dropping our carefully constructed wisdom so dramatically is a truth we don't like to admit to.

Information 'speed dating'

When we break the consultation into its component parts, the time we have available to give technical information is alarmingly small – perhaps only two to three minutes in a ten-minute consultation. By contrast, the information we have acquired over the years for each given condition is vast; we may have gone to day-long courses on a subject like diabetes – the Warwick Diabetes course, for instance, is five whole days of learning – and we are meant to distil this knowledge into an understandable precis of two to three minutes, tailored to the individual in front of us, mindful of guidelines to follow and safety issues that must not be missed. It's a wonder we ever get it right!

To help the trainees get used to this challenge, an exercise we would get them to do was what we called *information speed dating*. The trainees would get into pairs and each in turn would have exactly two minutes to explain a medical problem to the other; problems such as new onset atrial fibrillation, chronic obstructive pulmonary disease, coeliac disease and hypothyroidism were favourites. Each would raise its own challenges. For atrial fibrillation, is it helpful to explain what the atrium is? Should you describe fibrillation, and, if so, how? How do you explain the increased stroke risk? When do you start talking about anticoagulation? How do you explain why it might have happened? In their preparation for the CSA examination we would encourage the trainees to do the same exercise with a non-medical friend or family member, since we are often blind to our own use of jargon and sometimes we need a non-medic to call us out when we do this.

For each problem we are talking about, we might consider the following pyramid diagram.

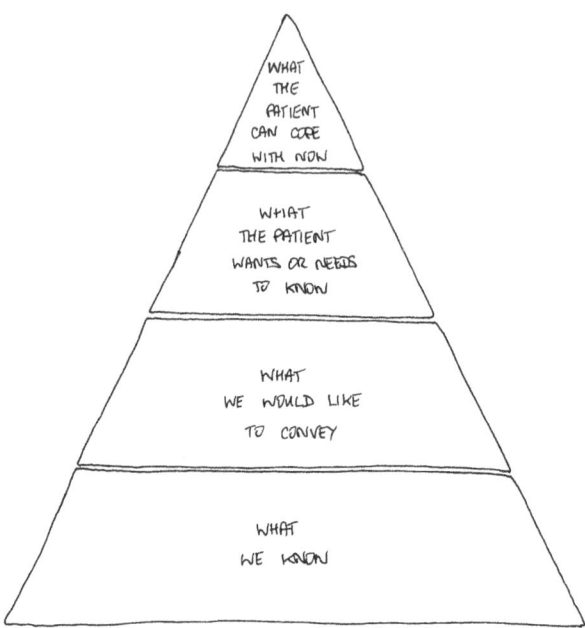

The doctor has a huge amount of knowledge, a proportion of which they would like to convey, but this is often not the same as what the patient needs to know, or would like to know. Most doctors have been attracted to medicine because they find it interesting, and there is a temptation to impart too much information just because we find it fascinating. Moreover, there may be information the patient does need to know, but it will be too much to give it all in one go and we need to break it down over more than one appointment – diabetes is a classic example here. Arranging to cover everything over two or three consultations can free the doctor from unreasonable time pressures and also give the patient the chance to think between appointments, return with questions and assimilate their understanding over time.

A question like "What do you know about asthma?" can sound horribly like a test

Of course, patients usually have some prior knowledge, which can give us a good head start, and enquiring about this can be a great way to start out in the High Tech Room. We should do this carefully, however. A question like, "What do you know about asthma?" can be well meant, but sound horribly like a test. "How much do you know about asthma?" is a less threatening way to start, leaving the patient the perfectly valid option of replying, "Nothing" without appearing stupid, but also leaving space for an unexpected reply such as, *"Well, I did my doctoral research on the role of interleukin 2 in the pathogenesis of asthma".*

Even when we have decided what information to impart, however, there is still the challenge of making it both understandable and memorable. The use of visual imagery can be very helpful here and we will consider this next.

Visual imagery

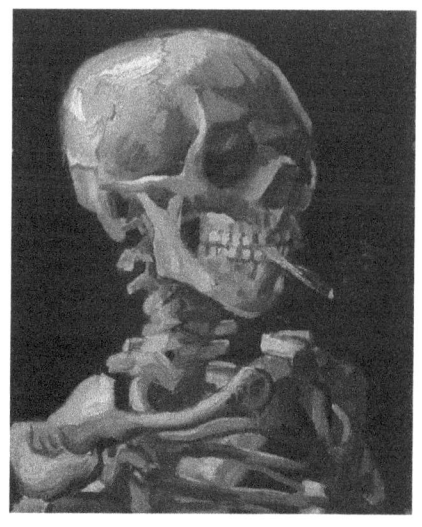

This small oil painting, *Skull of a Skeleton with Burning Cigarette*, is an early and little-known work by Vincent van Gogh. To modern eyes the painting packs a powerful visual punch – the lethal consequences of smoking are obvious at first glance. The joke was altogether different for van Gogh, however, since he was a lifelong smoker in a time before the health risks of smoking were known. Painted around 1885, it was probably a satirical comment on the insistence of the academic art world on painting skeletons as a means of learning anatomical structure. Van Gogh found the lessons uninformative and boring, and his sense of mischievous ennui comes across well with the amusing placement of the lit cigarette.

Even though the meaning of the image has changed over time, the fact that a picture can be a useful tool for getting messages across is clear, and something that we can use in healthcare. Just like all the other tools in our toolkit, the way we describe and explain medical problems can be tried, tested and refined depending on how effective our explanations seem to be; building up a working repertoire of visual images for different conditions can be extremely useful.

We should never be afraid to borrow these images from other practitioners, and one of the most powerful pictures I use comes from Tim Cantopher's excellent book on depression, *Depressive Illness: the curse of the strong*[1]. Cantopher describes depression as being like a bath with the tap running and the plug out, so that all the water is constantly draining away. He imagines taking an antidepressant as like

1. Cantopher, T. (2012) *Depressive Illness: the curse of the strong*, 3rd edition. Sheldon Press.

putting the plug in, but that this bath takes 2–6 weeks to fill. It is such a powerful image; in one short sentence it conveys and legitimises the feeling of emptiness someone may feel with depression, and explains how antidepressants don't work straight away, but should gradually help over a period of a few weeks.

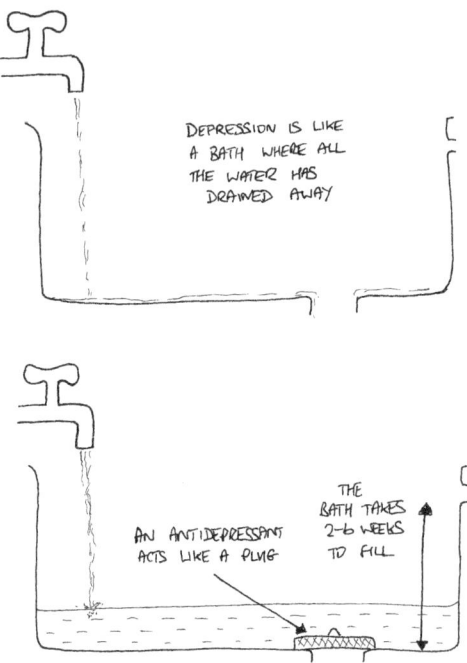

You can take the image further, explaining why taking the plug out too early will just cause the bath to empty again, and how making changes to what led to the depression in the first place is like shrinking the plughole so that in time the plug can be removed, but the inflow and outflow of water remain in balance. There are even ways to use the image for bipolar disorder, since we can consider that most people have an overflow in their bath, but that this may be blocked in someone with bipolar – explaining why an antidepressant can trigger an episode of hypomania. Mood stabilisers can be thought of as the old-fashioned plugs in school chemistry labs. For the uninitiated, these were a hollow plastic tube that fitted into the plughole, designed so that when the water level got to the top of the tube it would run down the centre and out of the sink, thus acting like both a plug and an overflow at the same time.

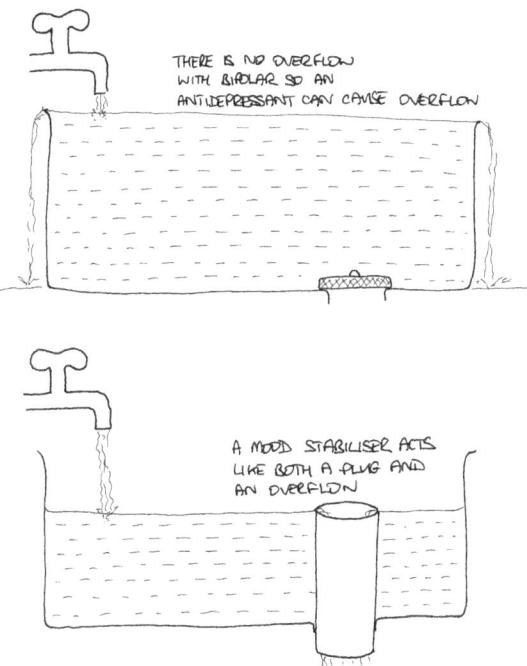

There are many other visual explanations that can make complex medical problems easier to both understand and remember. Some of the ones I have found to work are shown in *Box 10.1*:

Box 10.1 Visual explanations

Condition	Image
Depression	Depression is like a bath with the tap running and the plug out so that all the water has drained away (see above).
Benign paroxysmal positional vertigo	The inner ear has a spirit level in it so that we know which way up we are. Sometimes crystals get into the spirit level and then, like a Christmas snow shaker scene, they flurry up when we move our head, which makes us dizzy.
Burnout	Burnout is like a stress fracture. If you march 50 miles you might fracture your foot; you don't notice at the time, but the continual pounding means you can't even walk afterwards. Continual, pounding stress has this effect on our brain so that we suddenly find we can't function.
Carbocysteine (a mucolytic drug)	If we think of sputum like strings of spaghetti, carbocysteine chops it up into macaroni, making it easier to cough up.

Condition	Image
Explaining why we use cardiovascular risk to decide whether or not to treat hypertension or use a statin	Instead of quoting exact numbers, hold your hands up, palms together and about two feet apart. Say *"If your risk is this big, and we could make it this big* (move hands to one foot apart) *by taking a tablet every day, then you might be interested. Whereas if your risk is this big* (hold hands about 6 inches apart) *and by taking the same tablet every day you could make it this big* (3 inches) *then you might not be so keen."*
Kidney disease	Like a sieve that has got partly blocked up.
Protein or blood in the urine due to kidney disease	Like a sieve where the holes have got a bit too big.
Hypothyroidism – explaining why a *raised* TSH goes with an *underactive* thyroid	TSH is like the boss in the office; if the thyroid isn't working properly (hypothyroidism) then the boss shouts at it a bit louder (TSH goes up).

Of course, not everything fits into or needs a visual image to be explained, and some of the best images are medical diagrams or models which should also be in our toolbox (or on our desktop!). When we do use an image, we should decide if it actually helps, or just amuses us. You will find some of the examples I have described to be very helpful, but may decide that others don't add much to the explanation. We should do the same with every piece of information we impart – does it always help to know that insulin is made in the pancreas? Or that the thyroid is a gland in the neck? Are there phrases that are helpful even if they aren't visual? For instance, I have always found describing the bowel in irritable bowel syndrome as 'misbehaving rather than diseased' to be useful in getting over the essence of what I want to say.

Using jargon well

We often give trainees advice to *avoid* using jargon, and this is not bad advice, but neither is it complete. We cannot totally avoid jargon, and nor would we want to. How can we explain to someone that they have rheumatoid arthritis without using the technical diagnostic term 'rheumatoid arthritis'? What is more, there are times when a technical label can be very helpful and add value to our explanation. Telling someone that their rash is caused by a virus is a reasonable explanation, but when we can give it a name, like 'pityriasis rosea', we can use a piece of jargon to increase understanding. The diagnostic label provides validity to the patient's experience and increases confidence in our diagnosis – their rash has a name, and the doctor knew what it was (and the fact that our grand medical term 'pityriasis rosea' means nothing more technical than 'pink scaly rash' is neither here nor there!). The patient can now look up information about their condition based on the jargon term we have used, as long as we have explained it and used it in a way that empowers the patient rather than places us above them.

Empowerment, or avoiding disempowerment, is at the heart of using jargon well. Technical terms and jargon are always connected with power. They are designed to improve consistency by the use of clearly defined terminology, and to increase efficiency by applying a shorthand code (such as a diagnostic label) to a complex concept, but they inevitably touch on issues of power. Those who know how to use jargon are on the inside and so are more powerful than those who are unfamiliar with it. Our patients do not need to become fluent in medical speech to share in this power, but when we do use jargon, we need to ask ourselves whether we are passing power to the patient, or taking it from them. Using jargon without explanation is rarely empowering, and can frequently leave the patient feeling excluded from the conversation and disenfranchised, while using jargon well can empower the patient to understand their condition.

> **When we use jargon, we need to ask ourselves whether we are passing power to the patient, or taking it from them**

Using the patient's own language in favour of our technical terms can also help to empower them, as I was reminded recently when I went to buy a suit. Now suit-buying is a once in a decade activity for me and not something I relish. At one point, I wanted to find out if the suit I was looking at might develop those annoying bobbles that build up on wool clothing. Not knowing the technical term, I could only ask *"Is it likely to bobble?"*. The assistant was clearly very knowledgeable, having worked in the clothing industry for over a decade, and of course he could have used the technical word – 'pilling', I now know – but he replied *"It might bobble on the inside leg, but only after quite a lot of wear"*. Without any hint of condescension he knew what I meant and was very happy to use my word. This may seem very minor, but small actions such as this are the building blocks of good communication. In his case it helped him to sell me a suit; in ours it might mean the patient remembers more of what we say and is more engaged in the treatment plan we make with them.

Irregularly irregular

"I've looked at your heart trace and it does show that your heart has changed its rhythm and is doing something called atrial fibrillation."

The doctor paused for a moment, but was not surprised that her elderly patient looked nonplussed by this new information.

"It's very common, especially as people get older, and we have lots of patients who live quite happily with their heart doing this." She could see some of the tension drop from the man's shoulders. *"It means that the rhythm isn't as smooth as it is usually, which is why it feels like your heart is jumping about a bit."*

"It does that," he replied. He was a man of few words, but was listening intently.

"The other issue is that it makes the heart beat a bit too quickly. Yours is beating about 120 times a minute, which isn't very fast, but I think you'd feel more comfortable if it was less than 100."

"So how do we do that?"

"Well, we could start a tablet to slow it down a bit."

While the above example is certainly not perfect (the doctor made no attempt to discover prior understanding, for instance), it is a good example of how to use a technical term like atrial fibrillation, but to then explain it in plain English. The doctor covered what was most likely to matter to the patient (that it was common, you could live with it perfectly well and that it explained what he was feeling when his heart jumped in his chest), and avoided unnecessary detail (like irregularly irregular, or explaining what the atrium is or what fibrillation actually means). Of course, there is a place for explaining these details also; it might reassure the patient to explain that the atrium is the small, less important chamber in the heart and that the ventricle, as the main pump, is unaffected; or it might be that the patient has a good understanding of biology and would really like to know about the irregular electrical activity of fibrillation.

Watch your language

Hypos

This was the first diabetes review since Farah had started insulin, and everything seemed to be going swimmingly. The HbA1c was vastly improved and, by her own admission, injecting herself was not as bad as she had expected.

"Have you had any hypos?" the doctor asked, working his way down the on-screen template.

"No, none of those."

"That's good."

"But I get these terrible low-po's. I nearly passed out once and my husband had to make me eat sugar cubes until I came round."

Words are complex, and don't always carry the meaning we expect them to, especially within medical terminology. We have the Greeks to thank for the fact that our term for low sounds like high, but have we ever thought of the confusion that this might cause our patients? What is more, many words in everyday use have taken on a new meaning in the medical world and we have to be careful that we are not talking at cross purposes with our patients. 'Acute' and 'chronic' are typical examples: as a medical student I remember being completely thrown by the use of these terms and it took me weeks to understand them. Other than acute being the opposite of obtuse in geometry, I had no previous use for either word and there was no logical reason to expect that they referred to the timescale for a condition. More recently, the word 'chronic' has become commonplace in our language, but can mean something completely different to its use in medicine – a chronic headache might be used to describe a really severe headache, something more akin to what medics would mean by an acute headache! Or a patient might describe a severe headache as a migraine, but do they mean the medically defined pathophysiological process of a classical migraine, or the more colloquial use of the word meaning a headache that is worse than a more standard headache? We should also be aware that we are using such language as spoken word and not in written form, which opens the door for even more confusion; if we tell a patient that they had acute coronary syndrome, for instance, might they conclude that we are describing their coronary syndrome as cute? Not quite the meaning we intended!

Some commonly used medical terms appear to have the same meaning for both doctors and patients, but dig a little deeper and problems start to emerge. 'Blood thinners' is a good example. On the surface, it seems like a worthwhile attempt to replace the technical term 'anticoagulation' with a plain English alternative, and patients usually understand what we mean when we use it. All seems well, but I cannot be the only GP who has had patients ask me if their blood thinners are the reason they feel cold all the time, or get so tired. The problem is that telling someone that their blood is thin makes it sound like their blood is weak. We have expressions like 'blood is thicker than water' that reinforce our impression that thick blood is strong and nourishing, while thin blood sounds feeble and watery. What is more, the expression 'blood thinners' is not even medically accurate, since the blood is no thinner, just less likely to form clots. An explanation like *"It will make your blood less sticky"* may work better – who wants sticky blood?

> **I cannot be the only GP who has had patients ask if their blood thinners are why they feel cold all the time**

While it is easy to change our individual practice when it comes to a phrase like 'blood thinners', formal diagnostic labels are something we are stuck with and often throw us a curve ball when it comes to good communication – 'heart failure' is a classic example. This highly emotive term might helpfully convey the gravity of an end of life situation, but is likely to inappropriately terrify someone at the milder end of the 'heart failure' spectrum. Richard Lehman has long argued that the medical profession should change the term to 'cardiac impairment'[2] since the term causes such confusion, but the medical profession is yet to make the change and so we are left in a quandary. How should we describe it to patients? The word 'failure' will often appear in the notes and so we cannot avoid it entirely; impairment is certainly less emotive, but what does it mean? Impaired in what way? If we are to achieve a shared understanding with the patient, both terms need to be translated into plain English; *"Your heart isn't pumping as strongly as it should"* is far from perfect, but perhaps it is as good as anything.

The implications of some diagnostic terms go far beyond our own consulting rooms, but we are caught up with our patients in the confusion that surrounds them. Nickel *et al.*[3] argue that many cancer labels for low risk lesions – such as ductal carcinoma *in situ* (DCIS) and low grade prostate cancers – are misleading and result in overdiagnosis and overtreatment. The implications of this go far beyond the remit of a book on the

---

2. Lehman, R. (2005) Cardiac impairment or heart failure? *BMJ*, **331**: 415–416.

3. Nickel, B., Moynihan, R., Barratt, A. *et al.* (2018) Renaming low risk conditions labelled as cancer. *BMJ*, **362**: k3322.

consultation, but it is important to acknowledge the dilemma we are faced with in the High Tech Room when a patient has been diagnosed with DCIS and is faced with all the same treatment as a woman with invasive breast cancer. Do we explain that it is not really the same as breast cancer, and risk undermining her faith in the proposed treatment, or do we go along with the cancer label despite its misleading nature?

The scope of confusing medical terminology seems unending at times. In 2017, with the permission of the family involved, I wrote a piece for *BMJ Opinion*[4] about a very real-world problem with medical language I encountered in end of life care. The family of a dying patient were very clear that they wanted their relative to die naturally at home, but could not bring themselves to accept the term *Do Not Attempt Cardiopulmonary Resuscitation* (DNACPR). Hence we were entering the last days of life with no DNACPR in place, causing great stress to all the medical professionals involved! It took me a long time in conversation with them to understand where the problems lay with this familiar medical term. Eventually, I understood that resuscitation is far too broad a concept for what is intended to be a highly specific instruction about what to do when the heart stops – after all, don't we have an area in every Accident and Emergency department called 'Resus' where we do far more than simply perform CPR? The idea that we would *not even attempt* to resuscitate gave the impression that their much loved relative would be left uncared for if they so much as fell on the floor. *"Couldn't we just try?"* his wife said to me. In the article, I argued that *Do Not Perform Chest Compressions* would be a far better term; it removes any suggestion that we can't be bothered to try, and is limited to the specific (and appropriately unpleasant-sounding) act of chest compressions rather than the broader (and misleadingly humane-sounding) concept of resuscitation. Trying to change language in the world of medicine is a tricky business, however, and for the time being we are stuck with DNACPR, but at least we can use better language when we try to explain this unsatisfactory term, even to the extent of changing the wording on the form, which was what led to a satisfactory conclusion for my patient.

> **The idea that we would *not even attempt* to resuscitate gave the impression that a much loved relative would be left uncared for if they so much as fell on the floor**

4. Brunet, M. (2017) Let's ditch the word "resuscitation" in DNACPR. *BMJ Opinion*. Available at: bit.ly/37ZeOGS (accessed February 2020)

Conclusion

There is much more that could be said about this complex room. More than any, it is one where the doctor tends to take the lead, which allows us to practise and refine our explanations and bring our successes into the next consultation. However, the more the doctor leads, the greater the chance of leaving the patient behind; the doctor must be vigilant to make sure the patient remains with them at all times. Spending too long in this room can be as damaging as skipping it entirely, and the doctor may have to be prepared to come back to it two or three times in a single consultation, dealing in bite-sized chunks that the patient can digest. Ultimately, for complex issues, the doctor can also reassure themselves that they can return to the same room over time, helping the patient to build up a thorough understanding of their illness over several consultations.

Chapter 11

Optional Rooms

Pilates

After a busy morning winding a tortuous path through medically unexplained symptoms, complex frailty and a steady requirement for the tissue box, Dr Jones had nearly made it to lunchtime. Turning into the home straight always gave him a slight energy boost and he was further encouraged to find that his last patient had had the good grace to come with something straightforward: Mrs Watson had simple low back pain. Dr Jones had taken a good history; there were no radicular or red flag symptoms and he had even found time to ask her ideas, concerns and expectations; she thought she had tweaked it lifting boxes at work, wasn't too worried about it and didn't have any expectation as to what would happen next. As Mrs Watson hadn't yet thought to take any painkillers, the management was simple. Dr Jones performed a masterclass of safe prescribing, checking allergies, renal function and any past history of dyspepsia before prescribing non-steroidal anti-inflammatories with a proton pump inhibitor to protect her stomach. He explained the need to take it with meals, gave a clear set of red flag symptoms to watch out for as the perfect safety net, and advised her to come back in two weeks if she was still in pain.

As Dr Jones handed over the prescription, Mrs Watson looked troubled. Instead of putting it straight in her bag and thanking him, she held the piece of paper slightly at a distance as though it were somehow contaminated. *"I'm not really a pill popper,"* she said, *"do you think I'll still be able to go to my Pilates class this week?"*

We have all been Dr Jones at some point or other, where we realise we have surged ahead with a perfectly valid management plan, only to find we have left the patient behind without noticing, and that they have been too polite to warn us of the increasing distance between our positions until we have finally given them space to speak.

We have been taught to think in a one-dimensional way, with first-line, second-line and third-line options

The problem is that we have been trained to think History, Examination, Diagnosis and Management in a linear fashion, often only touching on the management plan once we are clear in our own mind exactly what the management should be. Even once we get to this last part of the doctor–patient interaction we have still been taught to think in a one-dimensional way, with first-line, second-line and third-line options and the implication that the patient should work through these in an orderly manner without being permitted to bypass one option in favour of another, or, worse still, to veto all the options we present to them.

I remember a very revealing discussion with a trainee who was faced with exactly Dr Jones' situation and was quite offended that his patient had requested physiotherapy without being willing to try analgesia first. He had an expectation that a person seeking medical advice should be willing to accept the advice given to them, and that physiotherapy was a finite NHS resource which should not be used lightly. There was some merit to his arguments, but there are many reasons why a patient might not want to take painkillers; perhaps they are especially susceptible to side-effects when they take tablets, or maybe they fear masking the pain and doing more damage, or they could just be sceptical about pharmaceuticals and prefer more 'natural' remedies. While the doctor may advise on the validity of these concerns, it is up to the patient to make the final judgement, and we certainly should not insist that a patient takes medication as a mandatory route to another treatment such as physiotherapy.

We have already discussed how the rooms in the *House of Decision* can be thought of as rooms containing potential management options, including investigations that might be arranged, treatments to be considered, referrals that could be made, or even a management plan as simple as a watch and wait policy. What many of the rooms have in common is that they are entirely optional – the patient may benefit from what is inside, but they will not take any great risk by missing the room altogether; a key skill in navigating the *House of Decision* is to identify such rooms, and check with the patient before entering them.

Analgesia in back pain is a clear example of an optional room. The patient may be more comfortable if they take painkillers, but they will not come to harm if they do not; stronger pain relief might be the prime purpose for booking the appointment in the first place, or the last thing on the patient's mind. Of course, all treatments are optional, since the patient can always withhold consent, but, as George Orwell might have said, *all treatments are optional, but some are more optional than others.* A good example of a treatment that is not really optional would be steroids in acute asthma; while many patients would not relish the idea of a course of steroids, the prospect of ending up in hospital, or worse, means the room with 'steroids' on the door cannot easily be bypassed. Indeed, the doctor may need to use particular skills to help the patient across the threshold of such a room, and these will be discussed in the next chapter – tackling Room 101. Rooms that are likely to be optional are common and extend far beyond painkillers. They include physiotherapy, much elective surgery, health screening, primary prevention of cardiovascular disease and much more. The beauty of these rooms is that, once they have been identified, they are easy to navigate in a highly time-efficient manner.

Open the door and take a look

The key to optional rooms is to take a look with the patient before deciding whether or not to venture inside. A simple question like, *"Would you like to talk about painkillers?"* or *"Would you like something stronger for the pain?"* avoids the possibility that the doctor will walk into the room and show the patient its contents in detail while only later coming to realise that the patient has politely waited in the corridor, with no intention of joining them. If the patient says, *"No, I can cope OK with the pain, thanks"* then both doctor and patient can move swiftly on. On the other hand, if the patient would like something for the pain, the truly shared decision is made to enter the room and find out more. The doctor can then describe the analgesic options, and ensure safe prescribing, in the knowledge that this is time well spent since it chimes with the patient's agenda.

Even within the room, there is still a need to keep the patient with us and not to get too far ahead. We can imagine the room marked 'painkillers' to contain three closed cupboards: paracetamol, non-steroidal anti-inflammatories and opiates, with the addition of an extra cupboard marked 'diazepam' for back pain with muscle spasm. Again, a quick look inside may prevent wasted time. *"How do you get on with codeine?"* may elicit, *"Oh, no, I felt so sick when I had that"* or *"I need to be able to drive, won't that make me sleepy?"* and so we are able to narrow down the options without going into too much detail first. Alternatively, the patient may be in a hurry to open one of the cupboards and the doctor needs to be the one to express caution. Thus, *"My friend said tramadol works really well"* might need to be met with, *"Yes, it can work well, but we do need to be careful with tramadol."*

The end result of entering an optional room might well be the decision to leave without utilising anything that was found inside. For instance, the idea of a painkiller might have been appealing to the patient until they heard more about the potential side-effects, but this is a perfectly good outcome, since what matters is that it was helpful for the patient to explore the room, and not time wasted while the doctor and patient are disconnected.

We might wonder why exploring the patient's expectations is not more helpful here. Returning to Mrs Watson, Dr Jones had taken the trouble to ask about expectations and received a neutral answer. The problem with expectations is, as has already been discussed, while they can be extremely helpful when the patient has a clear idea of what they would like to happen next, in reality this is the exception rather than the rule. For every patient with back pain who knows they would like to see a physiotherapist, there seem to be two or three that are not sure what they would like, or will not commit to stating their preferences, especially if they are asked too early. Moreover, when we ask the patient something like, *"Before I make any suggestions, did you have any thoughts about what we might do next?"* they are not likely to answer this in the negative and tell us what they do *not* want, and so they could be implacably opposed to painkillers, and yet make no mention of it when we explore expectations.

A patient who does not tell us what they want is not giving us licence to make the plan for them and expect them to do what they are told

This is not to say that we should ignore asking about expectations, but we should see it as a process of regularly checking in with the patient at the important points of decision rather than a single question to be ticked off when taking the history. When the patient tells us that they do not have any idea what we might do about their problem, that does not give us licence to make the plan for them and expect them to do what they are told; rather, it raises the skill level we need to utilise in order to help make a truly shared decision.

If taking too dogmatic an approach to optional rooms can jeopardise joint decision-making by leaving the patient behind, there is an equal and opposite trap doctors can fall into when it comes to optional rooms, which is for the doctor to abdicate their role as the expert who should guide the patient through the *House of Decision*. This is where the doctor throws open the doors to all the optional rooms at once and presents a range of options like a street seller laying out their wares, and asks the patient to take their pick. This failure of leadership can leave the patient floundering, and is a misinterpretation of shared decision-making, which is to be so afraid of patient autonomy that we don't share in the decisions and pass all the responsibility to the patient.

When considering optional rooms, we need to help the patient to understand what might happen if they choose not to enter. For our example of back pain the consequences will be obvious to the patient, in that they will need to cope with their level of pain, but for something like taking a statin in primary prevention of cardiovascular disease (CVD), the situation will be more complex, and require expert leadership from the doctor. Here the doctor and patient can still take a metaphorical look inside the room, but the patient may need some guidance before they decide whether or not to move on. The patient with familial hypercholesterolaemia and a CVD risk three times the average for their age will need a very different conversation to an older patient who has only just crossed the 10% CVD risk threshold where statins should be considered and has a lower than average risk. In neither case can the doctor simply ask *"How do you feel about statins?"* and move swiftly on if they get a negative response, since patient choice needs to be informed. On the other hand, nor does the doctor need to say everything there is to know about statins at the outset in order to steer the right course.

Some patients will ask the doctor to decide whether or not to enter an optional room. *"What would you do, doctor?"* or *"You're the doctor, I'll take your advice"* are common responses we might hear. How should the doctor approach this? In one sense, the patient has now given us licence to make the plan for them, and we will certainly want to consider the medical facts in their individual case and the guidelines we might choose to follow. However, even when the patient's choice is for us to take the lead, we still have an individual before us with unique preferences and priorities, and we can use our knowledge of our patient to help us make the best decisions. The patient may not be able to decide whether or not to take a statin, but they will be able to tell us how they feel about the risk of heart disease and stroke, and what they think about adding in an extra tablet. Some will have no qualms about swallowing as many pills as might be helpful, while others will feel the burden of medicalisation every time they go through the ritual of taking their daily tablets. One person may have a relaxed, fatalistic view of what might happen in the future, while another may be strongly influenced by their father's stroke and willing to pay the cost of being on medication to avoid the same fate. We can ask questions such as, *"How do you feel about being on tablets?"* or present the options in a way that helps them to contribute to the decisions by saying,

> **The patient may not be able to decide whether or not to take a statin, but they will be able to tell us how they feel about the risk of stroke**

"If what matters most to you is to avoid having a stroke and you don't mind being on tablets, then we can certainly give them a try, but if you ask me whether there is a really strong case for taking them then the answer is no."

We should certainly consider guidelines and best practice when we navigate optional rooms with our patients, but we must always remember that guidelines themselves are almost always more a group of options than a list of instructions. Most, in the small print that rarely makes the summary, state that patient choice is of vital importance, and use terms such as 'consider' or 'offer' to remind us that we must work with our patients, and that the missing ingredient in every guideline we consult is the opinion of the patient sitting before us. As Sir David Haslam, the former chair of the National Institute for Health and Care Excellence (NICE) once said, they are guidelines, not tramlines.

Box 11.1 Principles and tools to use when navigating optional rooms

Principles for gauging the patient's views before entering an optional room	Use your medical knowledge to work out which rooms are optional, and which are not
	For all rooms it is helpful to find out what the patient thinks about them, but with a truly optional room try to find out what the patient thinks about it before deciding whether to go in, or to safely move on
Tools to use when approaching an optional room	*"Would you like to talk about painkillers?"*
	"How do you feel about antidepressants?"
	"If someone offered you an operation to take this problem away, what would you say?"
	"Before I make any suggestions, did you have any thoughts about what we might do next?" (There is still a place to ask about expectations, just don't stop there if you get a negative answer!)
Principles for when the room is optional, but there may be consequences both for going in, or staying outside	Help the patient to understand what could be the consequences of missing out on this room: What could go wrong? What might they miss out on? Or if they are keen to proceed with a treatment or investigation that might have negative consequences, what might they be?

Tools to use when exploring how optional a room might be	*"We certainly don't have to use an anticoagulant, but if you want to reduce your risk of stroke then it is the best treatment for that"*
	"I think it's fine to delay a hip replacement at the moment, but do make sure you can stay active, as I worry when older people stop moving about"
	"We can certainly arrange a PSA test, and you might well be pleased to know if your prostate is OK or not, but it's important that you know that it might also lead to unnecessary treatment"
Principles for when the patient asks you to decide	Use your knowledge of their unique situation and medical guidelines to inform your decision, but also try to find out what is important to the patient, or how your suggestions might fit into their lifestyle
Tools to use when the patient asks you to decide	*"How do you feel generally about taking tablets?"*
	"If we use tablets we wouldn't be trying to make you feel better, we'd be trying to reduce your risk of having a stroke; how important is that to you?"
	"I think counselling would be helpful, but it does involve quite a bit of commitment – is that something you would be able to find the time for?"
	"We can certainly treat your blood pressure with tablets. Ideally it would be best to manage it with losing weight and getting a bit fitter, but could you see that happening at the moment?"

Chapter 12

Room 101

Custard

One of my favourite teaching sessions on the Guildford GP Training Scheme involved custard. The person leading the session would add water to a large mixing bowl, mix in custard powder and then choose an unsuspecting trainee to come forward and don an apron. The trainee would then be asked to make a fist and punch down hard on the liquid custard mixture. Remarkably, even when the Programme Directors stood well back 'so that we don't get splashed', the disbelieving trainee usually trusted us enough to go through with it and, of course, no splashes occurred. As their fist made contact with the liquid the pressure from the punch instantly changed the liquid's physical properties, making it behave like a solid; the experience is more like punching damp putty. As a physical material it is great fun to play with, since you can roll it into a solid ball that liquefies as soon as you stop rolling; you can even walk on it, and there are plenty of videos online of people filling a swimming pool with it and doing just that, yet sinking as soon as they stop walking.

Custard powder (or, more correctly, the starch in the custard powder) mixed with water has been given the fabulous name 'oobleck', a wonderful neologism created by Dr Seuss in his 1949 publication *Bartholomew and the Oobleck* where the hero has to rescue everyone from a green sticky substance that is gumming up the kingdom. Oobleck is a non-Newtonian fluid, which means its viscosity can change when pressure forces are applied to it, whereas the only factor that can influence the viscosity of a Newtonian fluid is temperature. Oil is a classic example of the latter, while ketchup, toothpaste, petroleum jelly and even blood are other examples of non-Newtonian fluids. Of course, if you keep adding water to oobleck it will lose this remarkable property, and if you want to try this experiment at home (I would thoroughly recommend it, especially if you have children!) then you must get the proportions right: the recipe is 200 g custard powder to 150 ml of water.

The point of teaching the trainees in this way is to leave them with a memorable image of something hardening under pressure, with the take-home message that, just like oobleck, if our patients start to resist what we are trying to do with them, then the harder we push the more they are likely to resist. We taught this as part of a session on motivational interviewing[1] (MI), to illustrate the first principle of MI, which is to roll with resistance. Traditionally, MI is used to help enable behavioural change such as smoking cessation or alcohol reduction, but resistance is not confined to these classic examples and will frequently be encountered in all manner of consultations. Sometimes, resistance is encountered with such force that it derails an important management plan; when that happens it is likely that we are standing outside the door to Room 101.

Sometimes, resistance is encountered with such force that it derails an important management plan; when that happens it is likely that we are standing outside the door to Room 101

Room 101, of course, was invented by George Orwell in his dystopian novel *Nineteen Eighty-Four*. The room is the ultimate torture chamber in the Ministry of Love and has the horrific quality that its contents relate to each individual's greatest fear; in the case of Winston, the book's unfortunate protagonist, this is to be attacked by rats, and the room quickly breaks his spirit. As doctors, we clearly never set out to torture our patients, but some of the tests and treatments we propose can feel close to torture, or at least the idea of them can tap into deep-seated fears in our patients. We should not be surprised, therefore, if we frequently meet resistance to our suggestions.

Unlike the omniscient Party in Orwell's novel, we do not have foreknowledge of our patients' fears. We can anticipate that some scenarios might be more stressful than others, such as an emergency hospital admission or the prospect of major surgery, but part of the joy of general practice is the rich variety of personalities we encounter; one patient will cheerfully accept our urgent cancer referral without batting an eyelid, while another will faint at the very idea of a blood test; one will seem unfazed by the awful complications they may encounter with chemotherapy, while another will be concerned about side-effects of any medicine we try to prescribe. One of the most important skills any healthcare professional must learn is to recognise the signs of resistance in the patient, to know when to back off completely and when to step back and work with the patient to overcome their resistance so that they can proceed; in short, we need to learn how to identify and navigate Room 101.

1. Miller, R. W. and Rollnick, S. (2012) *Motivational Interviewing*, 3rd edition. Guilford Press.

Identifying Room 101

A sticky problem

Dr Hon listened carefully to the whole story and asked the extra questions she knew she ought to ask, but from the first minute she knew what she had to do; as soon as he mentioned that meat was getting stuck on the way down it was clear that she would be doing a Two Week Rule cancer referral to investigate oesophageal cancer. Mr Jackson didn't seem worried about it – even the recent weight loss he put down to things being a bit hectic lately. *"So if you can just give me something for it,"* he said, after she had completed her examination, *"then I'll be on my way and won't bother you any more."*

"I'm a bit worried about it, actually," Dr Hon began, and then she explained carefully why she thought it might be cancer and how the urgent referral would work.

"Oh, I couldn't possibly do that!" exclaimed Mr Jackson.

"Why not?" asked Dr Hon, taken aback.

"I'm off to America next week, holiday of a lifetime. No, I can't possibly do that."

Room 101 is the opposite of an Optional room in the *House of Decision*. Whereas Optional rooms should be considered, but can be safely and quickly bypassed if the patient has no interest in them, Room 101 always contains something important which could be hazardous to ignore, or even life-threatening. Examples would include emergency hospital admission for suspected sepsis, steroid treatment for severe asthma, or an endoscopy to investigate worrying dysphagia. There is a more minor end to the spectrum as well, such as undertreating something like gout and the risk of accumulated joint damage over time; the stakes are lower, but the principles are the same. The other defining feature of Room 101 is that the patient is reluctant to venture inside. If the patient is fully on board with the decision then the room is simply an easy shared decision with a simple outcome, for instance:

> **Room 101 always contains something important which could be hazardous to ignore**

Doctor: *"I'm quite worried about how unwell you are; I think it might be an infection we call sepsis."*

Patient: *"I do feel awful, doctor."*

Doctor: *"I'm thinking you would be best in hospital."*

Patient: *"Yes, whatever it takes to get better."*

The decision to admit cannot be ignored, but there is no resistance and the encounter is straightforward. Yet the same encounter could take a different turn:

Doctor: *"I'm quite worried about how unwell you are; I think it might be an infection we call sepsis."*

Patient: *"I do feel awful, doctor."*

Doctor: *"I'm thinking you would be best in hospital."*

Patient: *"Oh, I can't go into hospital, doctor, not that."*

The doctor has now met resistance, and what seemed a simple room of decision has become Room 101.

The first challenge with Room 101, therefore, is to spot the signs of resistance. This may be non-verbal with a change in the patient's facial expression or body posture, or an involuntary shake of the head; or they may be more overt in what they say. When patients are reluctant to go along with our plan they often speak in absolute terms, using language such as *"I can't do that"* or *"I don't want those"*; in reality they will usually be more ambivalent than such statements suppose, since a degree of ambivalence is usually present in all human decisions. The skill of the doctor is to recognise the resistance inherent in such statements, but also not to be put off by their seemingly closed nature.

To enter or not to enter?

Once resistance has been recognised, the next question for the doctor to ask themselves, is just how essential it is to enter this room. When I was a medical student there was an older vascular surgeon who was renowned for being a highly trusted and competent surgeon, but not one who minced his words. The story went that a patient with a ruptured aortic aneurysm once asked him:

"What are my chances, doc?"

The surgeon considered, only for a moment: *"If I operate? Fifty-fifty."*

"And if you don't operate?" asked the anxious patient.

"20 minutes," came the reply.

Not all decisions are going to be as stark as the one this patient faced, but some will carry serious consequences if the room is ignored, while others may be much more open to negotiation. Declining surgery for a strangulated inguinal hernia, for instance, is unlikely to end well, while turning down a colonoscopy to investigate a change in bowel habit will usually do the patient no harm, since most patients with this symptom will not have a serious cause; there is a risk of missing cancer, of course, but this may be a risk the patient is willing to take. Deciding whether or not to start treatment with a statin is even more open to personal preference; the guidelines might say the patient should be offered one, but for the patient to choose not to accept it remains a perfectly reasonable option. When standing on the threshold of Room 101, therefore, the doctor needs to ask themselves some key questions:

1. How important is it that we enter this room? Should the doctor be encouraging them to go in, or is it reasonable to have an informed discussion in the doorway and choose to move on?
2. Who are we entering this room for? Is it to achieve what matters to the patient, or is it to allow the doctor to follow the guidelines?
3. What will be the consequences if the room is not entered?
4. How can the doctor help the patient to make an informed choice?

Crossing the threshold

We must never leave the patient floundering on the threshold of Room 101. If we find ourselves sounding like an exasperated parent asking their toddler, *"Well do you want it or not?"* then we are failing to show leadership. Neither must we bully them into the room, however, no matter how strongly we feel it is in their best interest to go

> If we find ourselves sounding like an exasperated parent asking their toddler, *"Well do you want it or not?"* then we are failing to show leadership

inside. The most likely outcome when doctors bully their patient is that the patient resists and all the doctor can do is to label them as difficult; on the other hand, the doctor may get their wish but even then there may be a more effective and supportive way to achieve the same end result. When we meet resistance, the most effective approach is to stop pushing, slow down what we are trying to communicate and listen more. There are several steps to this approach.

Step 1 – Agree with the patient

One of the most helpful things to do on the threshold of Room 101 is to agree with the patient's fears, for instance:

> *"I know. A telescope test doesn't sound very pleasant, does it?"*

> *"It's very reasonable to be concerned about steroids"*

Agreeing with their fears legitimises the fear and allows doctor and patient to examine it together, rather than to have an argument regarding whether or not it is something to be worried about. Note how important it is for the doctor to actively side with the patient. *"I can see why you would be concerned about steroids"*, for instance, leaves the fear with the patient; the implication being that the doctor can see why *they* would be worried, but a more sensible person would know better. More often than not, siding with the patient when acknowledging their fear creates an environment where they can re-evaluate the initial fear, putting one foot into Room 101 in the process: *"Of course, I'd rather not have a telescope test, but if you thought it was really important... would they put me right out?"*

Step 2 – Ask about the reason for resistance

While there will be common themes, patients will each have their own unique reason for resisting a given treatment. When it comes to steroids, for instance, one will be worried about diabetes, another will be concerned about weight gain and a third will simply have heard that they can cause problems. A patient may have a friend who was on steroids and knew how unwell they were, or another may be an elite athlete and worried that they might end up with a doping violation. Having acknowledged the legitimacy of the fear, the doctor can find out more by asking questions such as:

> *"What worries you about going into hospital?"*

"How do you feel about taking tablets for blood pressure?"

"What would concern you about being on insulin?"

Having learnt more about the source of the concerns, the doctor may be able to allay the patient's fears by using their expertise and experience, tailored to the individual fear:

"It's very reasonable to be worried about taking steroids after what your wife went through, but she had to take them for a very long time, and I'm glad to say that we only need to use a 5-day course here"

"You're right to be concerned about driving and insulin, you would need to check your sugars more when you drive, but there's absolutely no reason why this should stop you driving."

Step 3 – Help the patient to balance their fears

Frequently, the reason the doctor is so keen for the patient to go into Room 101 is that they have fears for the patient if they do not venture inside. Without exaggerating such fears, we need to raise these with the patient and see how they sit in the balance with the patient's own fears:

"It does sound a bit strong to have to take a course of steroids; the trouble is that your asthma is really quite bad at the moment, and I'm worried that if we don't do that then you might end up in hospital"

"I think you are absolutely right to try to avoid having too many medical tests, I'm just a bit worried that there could be a serious problem like cancer underlying all this and I would hate to find that out in six months' time when it might be so much harder to do anything about it"

"It's very reasonable to not want to go to hospital, but I am worried about how you will manage tonight as you'll be on your own, and you can't get out of bed to get to the toilet at the moment"

Ultimately, the judgement on how to balance such fears lies with the patient. The doctor needs to be confident that the patient has the capacity to make this judgement, of course, but needs to keep working with the patient whatever they decide. If they would rather take the risk of not going into Room 101, the doctor cannot just wash their hands of them and leave them to it. Is there a similar room that might not be the ideal treatment or plan, but would be more acceptable? Could the doctor try treating the pneumonia at home even if the patient really ought to be in hospital? Could some simple blood tests provide extra information before deciding on the urgent cancer referral, with the patient happy to accept the short delay this would entail? Sometimes the doctor will have to express the degree of risk the patient is taking in quite stark terms; for instance, a patient with temporal arteritis who refuses steroid treatment would be taking a very real risk of sudden irreversible blindness and no doctor could ever agree that this was a reasonable risk to take, but we should never exaggerate the risk, or imply that any patient who does not follow all of our advice is being irresponsible.

Step 4 – Leave the door to Room 101 open

Time has a habit of changing how we feel about things. I remember doing an advanced care plan with a patient once. She was clearly dying from an aggressive cancer, but wasn't ready to admit this; the cancer had progressed more quickly than anyone had expected and she was still catching up with events. We talked about cardiopulmonary resuscitation (CPR); to me, this was clearly a bad idea, but to her removing the possibility of CPR felt like giving up and we wrote a care plan recommending full active treatment. It was only a week later that I visited her at home. She was weaker, but most of all she had caught up emotionally with where she was physically; the previously frightening prospect of end of life care seemed now to offer her more hope than the hospital and we were able to completely rewrite her care plan so that she had a comfortable death at home. I could have insisted the first time that CPR was inappropriate and that as a medical intervention, it was a medical decision and not a patient choice, but it felt much more respectful of her wishes and dignity to make such a decision when she was ready for it.

Sometimes patients will never enter Room 101, but others may just need time or a change in circumstances before they are ready. We should aspire to give patients this time where we can, aim to always keep the door open and be prepared to revisit the room when we need to.

Box 12.1 Principles and tools to apply to Room 101

Principle: find areas of agreement	Agree with the patient wherever you can – it will help to empower them and encourages joint thinking
Tools to emphasise common ground	*"You're right, steroids are not something to consider lightly"* *"Like you, I would never want to have an operation without good reason"*
Principle: try to find out why the patient is wary of Room 101	Try to understand the particular concerns of the patient
Tools to help increase understanding	*"What would be your main concern about taking blood pressure tablets?"* *"Tell me what you think about taking tablets for depression"*
Principle: help the patient explore their own thinking	Share dilemmas and explore ambivalence
Tools to help explore thinking	*"As you say, methotrexate is a strong treatment, but my worry if we don't look after your joints properly is that you might end up with hands like your mother had"* *"I can see why you are reluctant to take them, but you also said you don't want to carry on like this"*
Principle: share your concerns with the patient	Use powerful words like 'worry' to help the patient understand the situation
Tools for sharing concerns	*"My worry if we don't refer you now is that we could really regret that in a few months' time if this is something serious"* *"I am quite worried about this"*

Chapter 13

Empty Rooms, Hidden Rooms and Locked Rooms

Tackling the Empty Room

In the year 63 BCE, the Roman General Pompey laid siege to the temple in Jerusalem. Having taken advantage of the Jewish Sabbath in order to assemble his battering rams outside the temple walls when the defenders could not oppose him, he brought down the outer walls the following day and his army destroyed any Jewish resistance, making Jerusalem a tributary of Rome in the process. The first century scholar Josephus records one of Pompey's most notorious actions on that day:

> "No small enormities were committed about the temple itself, which, in former ages, had been inaccessible, and seen by none; for Pompey went into it, and not a few of those that were with him also, and saw all that which it was unlawful for any other men to see but only for the high priests."

Josephus was referring to the *Holy of Holies*, that part of the inner sanctum of the temple which the Jews believed housed the presence of God. This small space was so holy that it was strictly forbidden for anyone other than the High Priest to venture beyond its heavy curtain. Even this high-ranking official was only permitted to enter the Holy of Holies on one special day of the year, the Day of Atonement. The Jews were so concerned not to violate this restriction that tradition states the priest would have a scarlet cord tied to him, so that if he were to be struck dead in the presence of God, his body could be recovered without anyone else having to enter this sacred place.

We can only speculate as to why Pompey chose to perform his infamous act of desecrating the temple by entering the Holy of Holies, but perhaps we need to look no further than a basic human instinct: the more our access to somewhere is denied, the more we want to break in, and the more hidden and exclusive somewhere appears to be, the more we want to be on the inside and not left out in the cold.

There was a meme on Twitter for a while where people would tweet something like, *"Hi, I'm a [insert your occupation here]. You might know me from some of my greatest hits like:"* followed by a list of phrases that such a person might frequently use in their job. It only lasted a few days and was hardly the most amusing or revealing of events on social media. What did interest me, however, was the number of GPs who stated that one of their frequently used phrases was, *"You don't need antibiotics."* It was usually antibiotics, but sometimes an MRI scan, and proved popular with other GPs who replied, liked or retweeted it. I noticed it because it is a phrase I have seen trainees use again and again over the years, and it rarely ends well.

What is wrong with saying *"You don't need antibiotics"*? As a statement of fact, it is correct – with a viral infection, of course, antibiotics have nothing to offer and it is important that GPs are judicious in their antibiotic prescribing. Some patients will be fully happy with this explanation; relieved even, since many patients are simply looking for an understanding of their symptoms and would rather not subject themselves to a course of treatment. What of those, however, who were hoping for a cure? What do they hear when we say, *"You don't need…"*?

Whenever we communicate, there are three levels of meaning that we usually portray:

1. The actual, obvious or literal meaning of the words we are saying
2. Hidden meanings that we have not stated overtly, but we have implied, and are probably aware of
3. Unintended meanings that the listener may infer, but we have not intended and are not conscious of.

For instance, if I'm talking with a friend and say something like, *"Oh, Steven, he drives a Porsche you know,"* the meanings may come across as follows:

1. The simple fact that Steven does indeed drive a Porsche
2. The unstated, but intended implication that I think he is a bit flash
3. The possibility that my friend could infer that I have a chip on my shoulder about Porsche drivers.

So, what meanings might come across with the statement we are considering about antibiotics?

1. The simple fact that they don't need antibiotics to get well
2. The implication that they are somehow not sick enough, or deserving enough, to have earnt access to this scarce resource
3. The unintended message that I think they have wasted my time.

For someone who was hoping that antibiotics might be the route to getting better, there are problems with all three of these meanings. Even the face value statement is problematic, for what do we mean by 'need'? I don't ever need to go out to a restaurant for dinner, since I can easily fulfil all of my nutritional requirements at home, but I still like to eat out once in a while – so there are things that I might still want, even if I don't *need* them. The patient may hear that they do not *need* to take the antibiotics to recover, but they might still hope to recover faster if they take them. In failing to state unequivocally whether or not there is any value in the antibiotics, therefore, one of the problems with the word 'need' is that it leaves the door open to the possibility that the treatment might still be beneficial.

The second, hidden, meaning behind the statement is the one that causes the most problems, since it implies a value judgement on how impressed the doctor is with the patient's illness. When the patient hears the statement *"You don't need antibiotics,"* they may hear the emphasis on the word 'you', implying that someone else would be more deserving of treatment. If we imagine 'treatment with antibiotics' as being one of the rooms in the *House of Decision*, we can consider ourselves in the corridor outside this room. Having listened to the patient, examined them and concluded that their infection is viral, we know that this is the wrong room to enter; it is empty, since antibiotics have nothing to offer them. When we utter those words *"You don't need antibiotics,"* we are effectively standing in the way of this room with our hand on the handle and our foot against the door. The word 'need' has neither opened nor fully closed the door but left it tantalisingly ajar with the light of the glittering treasure of a cure shining through the crack – treasure that is only available to those whom we have deemed *do* need antibiotics, an exclusive club to which our current patient does not have membership.

> When we utter the words *"You don't need antibiotics,"* we are effectively standing in the way of this room with our hand on the handle and our foot against the door

Is it any wonder that some of our patients, like General Pompey, set their feet firmly in the corridor and start to assemble their siege engines, determined to batter the door down? The first signs of the battering rams being in place can be, *"But my throat is so sore, doctor"* or *"But I've been coughing for nearly two weeks."* These are understandable attempts to convince the doctor that they really are deserving of treatment and can lead to escalating tensions as doctor and patient start to wrestle over the door handle to the room. The signs that the siege is really underway may include circumnavigating the guard at the door by finding another doctor, shouting at the reception staff on the way out or even making a formal complaint. All of it is stressful for both patient and doctor. One solution to this stress is simply to give in at every turn and prescribe antibiotics whenever patients ask for them, but clearly that is not the answer!

The issue for some patients is not that they want antibiotics per se, since there is nothing inherently desirable in taking a course of antibiotics (like there might be with controlled drugs, for instance). The patient has come to the surgery fed up with their symptoms and in hope of a cure; they might be interested in gaining some understanding along the way, but their intended destination in the decision-making process is to find a solution, and their prior understanding of the *House of Decision* is that the room marked 'antibiotics' is their best hope of achieving this. The challenge for the doctor is how to handle a room that they know to be empty, when the patient believes it to contain the solution they are looking for.

The best answer is to head for that room, take the patient metaphorically by the hand and head inside, showing them, with understanding, that the room is disappointingly empty. While it is hardly the equivalent of telling someone they have cancer, there is an element of breaking bad news here; the easy fix they were hoping for doesn't exist. We have to help them to understand this while ensuring we don't leave them feeling stupid or patronised in the process. A phrase such as, *"The problem with antibiotics is that, in your case, I don't think they will make any difference at all…"* might work well here. It is clear that there is no question of antibiotics helping, and, most importantly, it lacks any value statement: the emphasis is on whether or not the antibiotics will work rather than what the patient needs or deserves. It can be helpful to acknowledge the fact that it is reasonable that the patient might be so fed up with their symptoms that they are looking for a cure, with phrases like, *"Your throat looks OK, but that just means you don't have tonsillitis, it doesn't mean it's not very sore"* or *"Viruses can be miserable, can't they?"* This can help to validate the patient's concerns and defuse the arms race that can occur when the patient states repeatedly how bad they feel, and the doctor reiterates what they do or do not need.

The word 'need' is one to use with extreme caution in the consultation, but it is not without its use; it can be considered a 'power' word in that it conveys a value judgement that brings emotional power with it, for better or worse. At times, this power can be used to the advantage of both the doctor and the patient. For instance, there are often rooms in the *House of Decision* which the patient is aware of, and they are hoping to avoid, for instance the possible need for a hospital admission, or a referral for unpleasant-sounding tests. Sometimes these rooms have to be entered (see *Chapter 12* on entering Room 101), but often they can be safely left undisturbed. Clearly the doctor needs to do some groundwork by asking overtly what the patient thinks about these options, using prior understanding of the patient's preferences to guide them or paying careful attention to cues, so that they don't misjudge the situation. Once a shared understanding has been achieved, however, the doctor can reassure the patient with something like, *"Well, I'm happy that we don't need to admit you to hospital"* or *"I don't think a telescope test is necessary here"*.

Making use of Hidden Rooms

Having navigated the empty room, it is important to consider where to head next. The patient is still hoping for a solution, and we don't want to leave them staring at the four empty walls of the room marked 'antibiotics'! Sometimes hidden rooms can be helpful here, if we can find them.

A hidden room is a room that has something to offer the patient, but that they are either completely unaware of, know about but have forgotten, or know only in part. We might consider them like the hidden passageways in an old manor house – the false bookcase that opens to reveal an anteroom, or the door-shaped section of wallpaper with a keyhole hidden within its intricate design. If we can move seamlessly from the disappointment of the empty room into somewhere more hopeful then the patient, far from being fickle in some apparent love of antibiotics, will usually follow us, consistent in seeking something that might help. In the case of a prolonged cough, that room might contain treatment for the asthma that they have made light of, or the suggestion that their cough might

> If we can move seamlessly from the disappointment of the empty room into somewhere more hopeful, the patient will usually follow us

relate to reflux and the option of trying a proton pump inhibitor. It might simply include good tips that can help a viral cough – such as getting out of the cough cycle, sleeping propped upright, asking the pharmacist for codeine linctus or giving medical approval to a hot toddy!

As GPs we get very used to coming up with something to suggest for most things, and we quickly learn which are embedded in the popular imagination, and which are less well known. Suggesting to parents that they might give their child paracetamol for a fever is not bad advice, but they have usually got there before us; suggesting someone with a sore throat gargles with soluble paracetamol is often more novel, while the idea of putting moisturiser in the fridge to soothe itchy skin – something my own GP suggested for one of my children many years ago – has the triple advantage of usually being a totally new idea, appealingly logical and easy to put into practice; I have never forgotten this simple advice as a patient, and have seen it go down well countless times as a doctor. These nuggets of new ideas are invaluable in the GP toolbox; they are the keys to these Hidden Rooms and over time we need to try them out, see which work, refine the good ones and throw out the bad ones. Often the best solutions are the ones the patient comes up with themselves, but it is hard to come up with something you know nothing about!

While this chapter has used the issue of antibiotics for a viral infection as the key example, it is important to note just how commonly we have to navigate Empty Rooms and can bring the patient into a Hidden Room. The vexed question of an MRI scan with back pain is another classic example. In entering the Empty Room, we might try any of:

> *"The problem with MRI scans is that they often don't tell you what is going on"*

> *"MRI scans are really good at telling if a slipped disc is pressing on the nerve in your leg, but we already know you don't have that, because your pain is all in your back rather than your leg"*

> *"The thing about an MRI scan is that you would waste time waiting for it to be done, and it's only really helpful if we are thinking that you would need an operation... I wonder, what are your thoughts about physiotherapy?"*

The last statement uses that fateful word 'need' – here banking on the idea that the patient certainly does not want an operation and will steer away from the idea of a scan if it is the route to something that they agree they do not need; the suggestion of physiotherapy then involves opening the door to the Hidden Room, and seeing whether or not the patient wants to take a look inside.

In considering Empty Rooms we need to recognise that the lay person does not usually have the same degree of medical knowledge as the healthcare professional and so they are often guessing about what the treatment options might be, in a manner that is entirely reasonable. Take painkillers, for instance. A patient will often be clear in their mind that they would like a stronger painkiller than they have tried already, yet after a brief enquiry the doctor discovers that paracetamol is proving to be ineffective, that they are on warfarin so can't really take a non-steroidal anti-inflammatory drug, and that they don't want anything that might constipate them or make them drowsy, so ruling out opioids. How is the patient to know that we have only three classes of analgesia, and are now clean out of options? Often it is only by explaining the three classes of medication we use, discussing the problems with each and acknowledging that this leaves us with a problem, that we can help them understand that the room marked 'stronger painkillers' is proving to be empty. Once we have acknowledged this disappointment together then, maybe, we can explore the Hidden Rooms of other ways to manage pain – recognising that such offerings will always struggle to live up to the non-existent painkiller that would have taken the pain away quite beautifully without side-effects.

There is, of course, the possibility that all the rooms in the *House of Decision* appear to be empty, and Hidden Rooms have proved elusive. The patient clearly wants to find a solution, and yet no solution can be found, or the patient repeatedly rejects all the solutions the doctor suggests. This is not uncommon in general practice, particularly with medically unexplained symptoms, and an entire book could be written on this subject alone. While there is no easy answer, probably the most useful things the doctor can do here are to share the disappointment, avoid blaming the patient and continue to listen to their story. A narrative approach can be especially useful, and I can strongly recommend John Launer's work for this scenario[1].

> **Sometimes the most useful thing the doctor can do is to share the patient's disappointment**

1. Launer, J. (2018) *Narrative-Based Practice in Health and Social Care: conversations inviting change*, 2nd edition. Routledge.

Locked Rooms

An unexpected headache

Lucy had just made an appointment for a pill check. It was a little irritating that she had to take time out of her day like this, just to say all was well and get her next batch of contraceptive, but while she was there it would give her the chance to ask the doctor about the odd thing that happened the other day. She had been at work, quite stressed if she was honest, and found that she couldn't read some of the words on the screen; it was as if a hazy splodge had been painted on one side of her vision. It was quite frightening at the time, but only lasted 20 minutes or so and then was gone. Had she had a headache after? Yes, she had in fact; she assumed that was because of how stressed she'd been.

The doctor looked more concerned than Lucy had expected and then, completely out of the blue, said she would have to stop taking the pill. But she was so happy on it, it was suiting her so well…

There are plenty of rooms in the *House of Decision* that contain perfectly good solutions, but for an individual patient might as well be empty, since the door is firmly locked, and they do not have the key. The usual cause of this is when the solution is contraindicated; it might be that you would like to try beta-blockers for anxiety, but there is a history of asthma, or an MRI scan would be helpful, but the patient has an old shrapnel wound that would make this too dangerous, or a history of focal migraine with the combined oral contraceptive, as in Lucy's case. The room might be locked from the outset, or there may be the added complication that the patient is happily benefiting from the contents of the room and is now told they must leave. Lucy's example is just that, and we can imagine her being escorted from the room marked 'combined oral contraceptive' and watching the doctor firmly lock the door as she leaves. What this feels like will depend on how strongly attached she was to that room, the acceptability of other options and how the doctor handles this challenging situation.

> We can imagine Lucy being escorted from the room marked 'combined oral contraceptive' and watching the doctor firmly lock the door as she leaves

As with so many of the rooms within the *House of Decision*, the key to managing the Locked Room is to recognise it in the first place and have an open discussion with the patient. It will often be helpful to share their disappointment:

> *"This is frustrating as the pill was clearly suiting you very well in other ways"*

> *"Unfortunately, we can't use ibuprofen as we don't want that stomach ulcer to come back"*

On the other hand, we don't want to so emphasise how disappointing it is that the room is locked that we imply that the contents of the room are some wonder cure only available to others. Clearly it would not be helpful to say:

> *"It's such a shame that we can't use beta-blockers for your anxiety, they would have been so helpful"*

More useful (and truthful, since there are few wonder cures in medicine!) would be:

> *"Unfortunately, we can't use a beta-blocker with your asthma, but they only have a limited role and there is a lot more we can do for your anxiety"*

As with so much communication in the consultation, it is always helpful to listen well to the patient and agree with them wherever we can. If we can acknowledge the dilemma together then we are much more likely to be able to find other solutions, and for the patient to be open to them – perhaps there is a Hidden Room to explore here?

The doctor also needs to be open to imaginative thinking. Is the room truly locked? Is it just a relative contraindication and the patient is more willing to take a degree of risk than the doctor expects? Is there a way to find the key to the room? For instance, we may feel that hormone replacement therapy is contraindicated due to a strong family history of breast cancer, but perhaps some advice from a geneticist could shed more light on the risk? Sometimes a room is locked by issues of confidentiality; a relative might contact us and want to act, but we don't have the patient's permission to share their record or make decisions without them. Could we obtain consent in order to unlock this room? Or could we find another way of addressing the relative's concerns without breaking confidentiality?

Box 13.1 Principles and tools to use in Empty Rooms, Hidden Rooms and Locked Rooms

Principles to apply when preparing for the Empty Room	Reduce any sense of the patient's embarrassment that they thought the solution in the room might work – never leave them feeling foolish
	Agree with the patient wherever you can and incorporate their ideas into what you say – it will make it more acceptable to them
	Using *we* and *us* in your statements can help the patient to feel supported and not left isolated with their problem
Tools to bring the patient into the Empty Room, while helping them to save face and not feel embarrassed for hoping there was a solution to be found there	*"The obvious question here is whether or not antibiotics will help"*
	"You are right that we need to think about the role of a scan"
	"Let's think about whether medication has anything to offer here"
Principles to apply when showing that the room is empty	Be factual and non-judgemental, being careful with the use of any value-laden comments
	Expressing your concern about a treatment can be a valuable way of helping the patient understand why it may not be the best way forward
	Use the word 'need' with care – it conveys a powerful message!
	Share the disappointment that the room is empty
Tools to show that the room is truly empty	*"The problem is, antibiotics aren't going to make any difference"*
	"If this is viral then the last thing your body needs right now is antibiotics"
	"My worry about a scan is that we could wait a long time for it, and it won't tell us anything we don't already know"
	"The problem is that we don't have a tablet that can calm you down, there and then, that isn't also horribly addictive"
	"It's frustrating that we don't have an easy answer here"

Principles to apply with Hidden Rooms	Give the patient time to grasp that the room they hoped for is empty, but don't leave them there for too long if there is a good Hidden Room to lead them to
	Make sure they want to find a Hidden Room – are they truly looking for a solution, or did they just want understanding?
	Offer a statement that implies hope of an alternative plan (such as *"I wonder if..."* or *"There is a lot we can do"*) and gauge reaction before proceeding too far, to make sure they are with you
	If the patient has already hinted at the Hidden Room (in which case it is not truly hidden), incorporate their ideas whenever possible
Tools to lead the patient to a Hidden Room	*"If your priority is to get rid of this cough, then an inhaler might really make a difference"*
	"I think you are right that the problem is that your back keeps affecting you like this; I wonder if seeing a physio would really help to strengthen your back"
	"While I can't cure your pain, there is a lot we can do about it"
	"You also wondered about talking therapy – I think that would be well worth thinking about"

Chapter 14

Forecasting the future

Throughout this book I have stressed that we should consider the consultation in terms of two main objectives to aim for, rather than a series of linear tasks to complete. And now I am about to contradict myself. We have arrived at one aspect of the consultation that is inescapably task-based: forecasting what might happen after the patient leaves. Fortunately, this one task fits neatly at the very end of the encounter, making it easy to remember when it should be done, and we have plenty of opportunity to hone our skills in this area and embed it into our practice, since we need to make a forecast in most clinical encounters.

We can think of forecasting like the porch we must visit once we have been around both houses, a place where we pick up our coat and umbrella before we head home. There are consultations where there is no need to consider what might happen next – perhaps someone has just come in for a form to be completed, for instance – but these are rare, and it should be as instinctive as putting our shoes on after visiting friends for dinner that we visit the Forecasting Porch before the consultation ends.

> **We can think of forecasting like the porch we must visit once we have been around both houses**

Of course, the idea that we should look ahead to what might happen next is not an original thought of mine; the credit for embedding this concept into medical practice has to go to Roger Neighbour, and his description of 'safety-netting'[1]. Since Neighbour first described safety-netting as one of the five checkpoints in the consultation in 1987, it has become so embedded in medical education that medical students are almost universally familiar with its practice – even if disappointingly few know of its origins. Undoubtedly it is one of his most important contributions to the consultation and has saved many patients' lives as well as doctors' careers by encouraging the doctor to think of what could go wrong.

---

1. Neighbour, R. (2015) *The Inner Consultation*, 2nd edition. CRC Press.

Neighbour encourages the doctor to ask themselves three questions at this point:

1. If I'm right, what do I expect to happen?
2. How will I know if I'm wrong?
3. What would I do then?

These are essential questions for us to ask ourselves, and the term 'safety-netting' has a great deal of merit: it trips off the tongue with ease, is simple to remember and focuses on the most important aspect of forecasting, by placing the emphasis on safety. Predicting what might happen next is not only about being safe, however, and the biggest challenge is not only to *think* these questions, but to *communicate* these thoughts in a meaningful way to the patient. Neighbour does comment on what to say to the patient, but does not go into much detail, leaving room to develop his ideas as we shape our practice.

Still coughing

"I saw a doctor on Tuesday – I can't remember who it was – but he said to come back if it wasn't getting better. I'm still coughing."

Dr Shah had looked at the young man's notes before calling him. He'd come two days ago with what sounded like a flu-like illness: sore throat, cough, fever. She'd seen a lot of flu this week. *"So how long have you had the cough for now?"* she asked.

"About a week."

"And the fever?"

"Oh, that's all settled now."

"And your throat?"

"Much better, but I'm still coughing. The doctor said to come back if I wasn't better in a couple of days."

Dr Shah sighed; it was going to be a long day.

Dr Shah is faced with an uncomfortable dilemma. The young man is clearly getting better but has an unrealistic expectation with regard to his cough; while two days was a reasonable timescale to review if he still had high fevers, his cough was more likely to last another two weeks. And yet, he had been told to come back in a couple of days if he wasn't better, so he was only following instructions. How is she now to re-educate him, without making out that either the patient or the previous GP is stupid? We've all been there.

If we think solely in terms of patient safety then Dr Shah's patient has certainly been kept safe, but there was clearly a gap in shared understanding between the doctor and patient when it came to what 'better' looked like. There are many examples of this: a sebaceous cyst that fails to go away; treatment with an antidepressant or a steroid inhaler that was abandoned after a few days as it wasn't helping; a mouth ulcer that still hurts after a week – all may lead to an unnecessary follow-up appointment, or a treatment plan that falls apart. Just as one of the primary objectives of every consultation is to achieve a shared understanding between doctor and patient, so a shared understanding of what might happen next is equally important, and we need to develop the skills to achieve this goal.

Communicating the forecast

Neighbour's three questions remain the key to making a forecast, and when it comes to sharing our forecast with the patient, there are four important principles to bear in mind:

1. Be specific

Advising the patient to 'come back if it's no better' is better than nothing, but not by much. As safety nets go, it is pretty threadbare and unlikely to be much better than what the patient would do anyway. Like most patients, the young man who came back to see Dr Shah had multiple symptoms, so which are the ones that matter? Which should he be taking note of, and on what timescale? It may be that we need to set different expectations for individual symptoms. More specific forecasting might look like this:

> "I think your sore throat will settle in the next few days, but I'd be concerned if you still had a high temperature in two days' time. Your cough might take another couple of weeks to settle, I'm afraid."

One of the challenges of being more specific, of course, is that there is more information to get across and so more danger that we might overload the patient so that they don't recall what we have said anyway. The above statement is a big improvement on just saying to come back if it's no better, but it has only considered the symptoms the patient has at the moment and not new symptoms that might arise. The doctor will need to at least pause to give time for the patient to digest what has been said, but could then continue:

> *"What would most concern me is if you started to feel a lot more poorly in yourself, or if you had any trouble with your breathing. I don't expect either of those to happen, so I would want you to see a doctor the same day if they did."*

Clearly, we need to avoid alarming the patient when we talk about what could go wrong, and the tone and manner of how we deliver our forecast is as important as the exact words we use, as is a knowledge of the patient we are working with. The use of a negative like *"I don't expect…"* is worth thinking about carefully, since, as humans, we often don't hear negatives well. My heart sinks when a well-meaning parent sits their child on their knee and says, *"It's OK, the doctor's not going to hurt you."*

> **My heart sinks when a parent says, *"It's OK, the doctor's not going to hurt you"***

I know that the only word now reverberating around the poor child's mind is going to be 'hurt', and this is usually confirmed by their tightening body language as I approach with my stethoscope. So, if I am going to use a phrase like *"I don't expect…"*, I need to be aware that what I don't expect may be exactly what the patient goes away remembering. This could be valuable and add emphasis to the safety aspect of my forecasting but could also lead to unnecessary heightened anxiety. As with so much of how we communicate, it is a judgement call; the use of negatives has its place, but we should proceed with caution.

2. Give sensible timescales

I remember seeing a child in the evening duty surgery a few years ago. She was about four years old and had already been seen that morning with a very straightforward viral infection; before I called her in, I was distinctly unimpressed that her parents had brought her back so soon. Were people so reluctant to accept the diagnosis of a virus that they have to get a second opinion *the same day*? When her dad told me she had a rash, I could at least see why they might have wanted to come back, but I still told myself that we needed to help parents get better at recognising non-specific viral rashes and to know that they are par for the course. It was when he showed me the dramatic bruising rash all over his daughter's legs that I realised how judgemental I was being: she had a particularly striking case of Henoch–Schönlein purpura and I arranged for the paediatricians to see her without delay.

When we set timescales for review, we must always create an atmosphere that gives permission for the patient to return sooner than we expect, because we must always be ready for the unexpected. On the other hand, to ask someone to return in two weeks if their ganglion is no better, or in two days if they still have low back pain, will clearly waste time for both the patient and the doctor. Trainees can find it difficult to set long timescales for review, and even more to say that something should not be reviewed at all, since it feels unsafe. There are some questions we can ask ourselves that may be helpful as we try to work out what timescales to suggest:

1. If the problem is unchanged, at what point (if any) would I suggest a different course of action? How can I communicate this to the patient?
2. What changes might happen that would mean the patient should come back quickly? And what do I mean by quickly? This could be anything from calling 999, to seeing a doctor the same day, or coming for a review that week; it's important to be clear.
3. Is there anything that might change from the patient's perspective that would make a review worthwhile? For instance, if they no longer need to care for an elderly relative, they might be ready for a knee replacement; or if they get fed up with their back pain, they might like to reconsider physiotherapy.

3. State what you expect, not just what you don't expect

When we think of forecasting as primarily about keeping the patient safe if things go wrong, it is easy to forget Neighbour's first question: *"If I am right, what do I expect to happen?"* It might not be important for saving someone's life if we neglect this aspect of forecasting, but it can be really helpful if we are able to communicate what we expect if we are right. This is particularly important when we expect something to NOT resolve, or at least to take a long time to settle. When we see a young child with reactive cervical lymph nodes, for instance, while we need to make sure that we see them again if the nodes get progressively larger, we will also need to convey that the nodes might always be palpable, or we will worry her parents when they can still feel them a week later. If we expect someone's tennis elbow to take weeks or even months to resolve then we need to prepare them for this, while also avoiding giving the impression that we expect the pain to be with them forever. For instance, we could say:

> *"It does take a while for tennis elbow to get better; it tends to be weeks or even months rather than days, but the actual elbow joint is fine so whatever we decide to do, I expect this to get fully better over time"*

This aspect of forecasting is especially important when it comes to medication. We have to try particularly hard with treatments that have no immediate effect, like antidepressants or a steroid spray or inhaler. We can even make a joke of this as a way of making it memorable:

> *"I'd like you to try a steroid nasal spray, but when you use it you won't feel ANY better at all at the time – 'Great!' I hear you say!"*

or

> *"The steroid spray is like the opposite of a decongestant spray; decongestants feel great at the time, but don't solve the problem and can even make it worse if you stay on them. With the steroid spray it doesn't make you feel any better at the time, but if you use it regularly then it will start to solve the problem."*

4. Check understanding

Checking understanding has always been a tricky area in the consultation. We know that it is important, and that misunderstandings are commonplace, but how do we do it efficiently? Classically it has been taught that we should ask the patient to explain back to us what has been agreed, or to ask how they will explain it to a relative. This certainly has its place, but it is cumbersome and hard to do without sounding patronising. How do we check understanding more efficiently?

The groundwork for ensuring understanding should have been done well before we get to the Porch. Remembering that the consultation is like a dance (see *Chapter 3*), if we have managed to 'stay in hold' in the dance then it is likely that we will have developed a shared understanding and been able to check it along the way. Staying in hold means being sensitive to verbal and non-verbal cues that warn us if the patient is losing touch with us, and checking in with them regularly as the plan unfolds: How do they feel about this? What are their thoughts on that? When it comes to planning an interval for review it may involve overtly handing over the decision to the patient by asking *"When would you like to come back to see me?"* The more the patient has helped form the decision then the more we can assume they have understood it. How we finish our basic sentences can also be important. There is a world of difference between asking *"Is that OK?"* at the end of a sentence compared with *"How does that sound?"* or *"How do you feel about that?"* The former can only be answered as *"yes"* or *"no"*, and it can be hard to tell a doctor that their plan is not OK, while the latter invites a fuller and more honest answer, including space for the patient to ask for clarification of something they have not understood.

> **The groundwork for ensuring understanding should have been done well before we get to the Porch**

Even with a truly effective shared understanding, however, there may still be some hard information we need to get across at the end of the consultation. There may be red flag symptoms for the patient to watch out for, explanations as to how to get help out of hours if needed, understanding about planned follow-up, tests for the patient to organise or details about when to come back sooner. It can all be a bit overwhelming. And even if the patient can rehearse the plan with us before they leave, that is no guarantee that they will remember it once they have left the surgery. Hard facts are often best remembered when they are written down, and a small degree of effort on the part of the doctor can make a big difference here. Whether it is writing a few points by hand and giving it to the patient, printing out our consultation notes as a summary for them to take away, or sending a text once they have left, our forecast will be significantly more effective if we can give them some form of written summary. Texting is particularly appealing when the system we use also puts the text into the patient's notes – what better medical defence than to have our forecast clearly entered into the notes in this way?

Box 14.1 Principles and tools to apply to forecasting

Principle: give a different forecast for different aspects of the problem	Be specific, with different directions for different aspects of the problem
Tools for being specific	*"I'd expect the tablets to help your heartburn in a couple of days, but if your cough is being caused by the reflux then that could even take a month or two to settle"* *"There are three things to watch out for with sciatica: any weakness in your leg, say you can't lift your toes properly for instance, any numbness in your saddle area – the bit of your bottom that would sit on a bicycle saddle – and any loss of control of your bladder or bowels. We call these red flags, and if you get any of those then you should see a doctor the same day."*
Principle: give sensible timescales	Be exact, use actual terms like days or weeks rather than vague statements
Tools for giving timescales – or circumstances that would change the situation	*"Back pain like yours usually settles within a week or two; sometimes it takes longer. If it goes on for four weeks or more then it is certainly worth thinking about something like physiotherapy."* *"I would expect the antibiotics to start working within two to three days, so give me a call if it is still stinging after that"* *"It's not a mild bunion, but it's not very bad either. I think we're agreed that you wouldn't want an operation at the moment, but if it gets more painful then you can certainly let me know and we can refer you. How does that sound?"*
Principle: don't just think about what might go wrong	State what you expect, not just what you don't expect
Tools for describing what you expect	*"With an antidepressant, if you feel any better at two weeks then that is a bonus. I'd hope at that point that any initial side-effects you might have had will have gone, and then I hope they will start to kick in between two and four weeks."* *"A cyst like this might get smaller and go away, but sometimes they just stay like this in the long term, in which case they are best left alone"*

Principle: check understanding	Avoid just asking if the plan is OK
Tools	*"How does that sound to you?"*
	"How do you feel about that?"
	"I've said quite a few things here, shall we just go over it to make sure we've got it right?"
	"Would you like me to send you a text to summarise the plan?"

Chapter 15

Putting it into practice

One of my frustrations with consultation models is the translation of theory into practice. A model that works well in one consultation may seem quite irrelevant when we are faced with an entirely different dynamic with the following patient. What might suit a consultation for a patient presenting with a new problem could have little to offer us when conducting a follow-up, or a medication review, or when faced with a list. Perhaps the boldest claim in this book is that the *Two Houses* model can apply to every single consultation; how well it achieves this is up to the reader to decide, but in this chapter I will attempt to demonstrate this claim by analysing three different consultations, with a commentary on what is happening in each interaction, and how this applies to the model. What is important to bear in mind is that the model is not a series of linear tasks that should be followed in order, but the twin objectives of achieving a shared understanding of what matters and deciding together what to do about it, with the two houses providing tools and structure along the way.

> **Perhaps the boldest claim in this book is that the *Two Houses* model can apply to every single consultation**

Each consultation will be written as an imagined transcript between doctor and patient, with accompanying commentary. Clearly this will not be an attempt to describe every word that would be said in the consultation, but an abridged version to highlight the interaction. We will start with a very simple consultation.

Scenario 1 – Paronychia

Patient: *"It's this finger, doctor, it's so sore!"* (shows index finger to the doctor, which has a clear paronychia with a tense collection of pus)

Doctor: *"Oh, that does look sore."*

The opening gambit includes a heavy cue that the patient may be looking for a solution in the *House of Decision* when she describes it as 'so sore'. By acknowledging this, and repeating the patient's own words, the doctor is signalling a shared understanding that pain is a problem, and hinting towards looking for a solution.

Patient: *"I can't have another night like last night."*

Doctor: *"I'm sure."*

"I'm thinking it looks infected."

Patient: *"Yes, that's what I thought."*

Doctor: *"I could easily use a needle to get that pus out."*

Patient: *"I'd been wondering about doing that myself."*

Doctor: *"It would make it a lot less painful."*

Patient: *"Then let's do it."*

The patient reinforces the cue by stressing how it affected her sleep the night before. This is the sort of consultation that is so simple that most doctors would dispense with tools like ICE, or summarising – it just seems foolish to ask the patient what they think when it is so obvious that there is infection. Instead of asking what the patient thinks is the problem, therefore, the doctor floats the idea of infection by stating what he is thinking, and achieves enthusiastic agreement with the patient. The cues have been strong enough to suggest going straight for the solution of releasing the pus, and agreement is easily achieved.

(after releasing the pus)

Patient: *"That feels better already."*

Doctor: *"That's good. We need to think about how to treat the underlying infection. It depends on how you feel about taking antibiotics. The quickest way to deal with it would be to have some antibiotics by mouth, but it might well settle with an antibiotic cream if you would prefer to avoid taking any medicines."*

Now that the immediate problem has been dealt with, treatment options can be discussed by reviewing them in the *House of Decision*. The doctor has approached two optional rooms, oral antibiotics and topical antibiotics, and helped the patient to decide which to enter by asking both *how she feels about antibiotics* and also *how quickly she wants to get rid of it.* By weighing these two factors, the patient is helped to make the right decision.

Patient: *"I just want to get rid of it, doctor."*

Doctor: *"Then let's go for a course of antibiotics"... pause... "Is the infection going to cause you problems, at home or at work, for instance?"*

Patient: *"No, not really. It's just so annoying."*

Once the patient's priorities are clear, the course of action is decided. The urgency with which she wants to resolve the problem is another cue that there may be an underlying reason why it is problematic to her and the doctor explores this. Had she been a gardener, or worked in a kitchen with constant hand washing, for instance, there might be the need for prevention measures.

Doctor: *"I would expect it to be a lot better within 2–3 days, so if it is not better, or if it gets worse before then... certainly if that pus comes back... then I would want to see you again."*

The doctor closes the consultation by forecasting, explaining what he would expect to happen and in what timescale.

Such a simple consultation can often seem too trivial to apply to a consultation model, and any linear model is often derailed when the patient immediately presents the doctor with a request to examine something as part of the opening gambit – since examination is usually meant to happen around midway through a consultation. However, far from becoming doctor-centred, by noticing cues and checking understanding the doctor can efficiently move to a shared plan, with the patient included at every stage.

The second scenario is a more complex initial presentation of a problem.

Scenario 2 – Dysphagia

Patient: *"I won't keep you long, doctor, I just need something for this swallowing problem of mine."*

Doctor: *"Yes, of course, what's happening?"*

The patient immediately declares the wish to find a solution to the problem in his opening gambit. By the simple reply *"Yes, of course"*, the doctor expresses a willingness to help *('popping the bubble')* and promises to visit the *Solutions* wing in the *House of Decision* at a later stage.

Patient: *"It's not much really, it's just that when I swallow... things get stuck about halfway down. Not everything, I can drink fine and soup's OK."*

Doctor: *"Mmmm... and how long's that been for?"*

Patient: *"About the last 2 months; I can't understand it."*

Doctor: *"Have you been worried about what it might be?"*

Patient: *"Gosh, no. I just want to be able to eat a good steak!"* (laughs)

The doctor picks up a cue that the patient *'can't understand it'*, implying that he would like to gain more understanding (and hence notes that she will need to visit both wings in the *House of Decision*). She follows up the cue by exploring concerns, but this is met by humour – does that mean he is not concerned, or does not want to reveal any concerns? At this stage it is clear that what matters to the patient is that he would like a solution to the problem and would like to know more about it. What matters to the doctor is that she is already worried that he may have oesophageal cancer, since food getting stuck halfway down is a red flag for cancer, and knows she will need to talk about an urgent cancer referral – she has *found dry rot*. She is already anticipating that there could be a Room 101 ahead and knows she will need to make time for this. After listening to more of his story, the consultation proceeds.

Doctor: *"There's a couple of things I just need to check. I know you don't smoke, what about alcohol?"*

Patient: *"Oh, I like a glass of wine."*

Doctor: *"Sure, what would be typical?"*

Patient: *"My wife and I share a bottle with dinner. I probably have more than she does. Is that a problem?"*

Doctor: *"Sometimes it can make digestive problems worse."*

The doctor indicates a trip to the basement by signposting that there are *"a couple of things I need to check"*. Alcohol is a risk factor for oesophageal cancer and so it is entirely relevant to ask about it, and she will go on to ask about weight – more interested in weight loss than obesity in this instance. After examining the patient, she knows there is more work to be done in order to achieve a shared understanding.

Doctor: *"This is clearly quite a nuisance for you, and we need to see how we can resolve it. I am a bit worried about what might be causing this."* (pause)

Patient: *"Worried?"*

Doctor: *"Well, when doctors hear that food is getting stuck, we worry that there might be something there getting in the way, and sometimes that can be quite serious."* (pause)

Patient: *"You think it's serious?"*

Doctor: *"Well, I don't know at the moment. Sometimes there's quite an innocent reason for food getting stuck, but what we need to be concerned about is that sometimes this can be caused by a growth in the food pipe, a cancerous growth. That's what we need to work out."*

The doctor indicates that she is still aware of the need to find a solution by acknowledging what a nuisance the problem is, but she has found *found dry rot* and knows that she may need to help her patient into Room 101. There has been no indication yet that he has thought of a serious cause, and so she prepares him for this room in stages, leaving pauses for the patient to respond before taking him further. Having achieved this she will then have a clear way of explaining that finding a solution is dependent on gaining greater understanding, and can explain how an urgent referral will achieve this. Having negotiated this, the patient returns to the issue of wanting a solution.

Patient: *"So can you give me something to help the food go down?"*

Doctor: *"Sorry, I did mean to come back to that. It is a tricky one. It would be very helpful if there was a tablet that would help. The problem is that I think it might be more of a mechanical problem that's stopping the food pipe from working properly and so I don't think there is a tablet for it."*

Patient: *"Oh."*

Doctor: *"That is frustrating. I think we need to know what is causing the problem before we can fix it. At least we know the hospital will see you quickly for this, so it shouldn't be too long before we know what we can do about it."*

With the emphasis on achieving a two-week rule referral, the doctor has forgotten the initial cue that the patient hoped to be given something that would help. This is common, since doctors are only human and we might signal a willingness to go to the *Solutions* wing, but get distracted on the way. The initial signal to the patient may still help them to feel able to bring us back to it, however. The challenge now is that the doctor is faced with an empty room; she could try something to suppress acid, but knows that if there is a physical problem like a cancer, or oesophageal dysmotility, then this will make little difference. She takes him into the empty room and explains the dilemma, while recognising the disappointment of not being able to give an immediate solution. The speed of a two-week rule cancer referral may be some compensation and operates as a hidden room in this scenario.

Before closing the consultation the doctor will need to forecast the future, placing the emphasis on what to expect with the referral, when to contact her if he doesn't hear anything and how to get in touch afterwards if he wants to talk over how it went.

What this scenario illustrates is how an opening gambit like, *"I just need something for my swallowing; food keeps getting stuck"* can give the doctor an immediate idea of the structure that needs to follow. Already it is clear that a solution is sought, yet the doctor can anticipate that the solution the patient has in mind might be an empty room; she knows that there is no quick pill for dysphagia and *"I just need something"* sounds like the patient is hopeful for a simple treatment that probably doesn't exist. What is more, since difficulty swallowing is a red flag symptom for cancer, she already knows that the likely outcome will be an urgent cancer referral. She will be uncovering 'dry rot' (see *Chapter 7*), since this will not be good news. The patient may already be aware of the possibility of cancer and relieved at the idea of a quick referral to find out what is going on, but the doctor also needs to consider that she might encounter resistance to the idea – in other words, such a referral could well represent a Room 101 and she will have to consider how to help the patient face this room.

To put it in the language of the *Two Houses* model, this is not a time for gardening

In order to navigate these quite tricky rooms effectively she will need to explore her patient's symptoms in more detail and also try to understand his own perception of what is going on. For instance, how strongly does he believe there is a simple cure for his symptoms? Perhaps more importantly, has he already thought that he might have cancer and his opening gambit is an attempt to make light of his concerns, or will the idea of a cancer referral come as a complete shock to him? However the consultation plays out, it is clear that the doctor will need to leave time for these rooms, and therefore she will have to be careful not to get distracted elsewhere. So, although a quick trip to the basement to find out about alcohol consumption is justified, this is probably not the time to start talking about other matters such as weight reduction or to check her patient's blood pressure – to put it in the language of the *Two Houses* model, this is not a time for gardening.

In contrast, the final scenario is a patient with hypertension coming for a medication review, a situation where the garden takes centre stage.

Scenario 3 – Blood pressure review

Patient: *"Just here for my review, doctor."*

Doctor: *"Great, anything to report?"*

Patient: *"I'm fine with the tablets. My knees are playing me up a bit."*

When someone comes for a review there are clear objectives for the doctor, but there is still a need to find out what matters to the patient and something like *"Anything to report?"* is an effective way of helping the patient to contribute to the agenda right from the start. The doctor discovers that his patient's knees are a nuisance, but, after exploring further, learns that they are not a major problem. He will come back to that later, but needs to conduct the review as well.

Doctor: *"Thank you for bringing in your home blood pressure readings. What did you think of them?"*

Patient: *"They're a bit higher than usual."*

Doctor: *"Yes, I thought that."*

Patient: *"I put a bit of weight on after Christmas; I expect that hasn't helped."*

Doctor: *"It can certainly affect blood pressure."*

Patient: *"Is it very bad?"*

Doctor: *"No, it's higher than I would like, but it's not very high. If it stayed at this level, though, we might need to consider adding a second tablet. How would you feel about that?"*

Patient: *"Well I would if you thought it was needed, but I'd rather not. Perhaps if I lost the weight first?"*

Doctor: *"Yes, I think that would be a good idea, it might help your knees as well."*

Medication reviews are often conducted in the garden, and here the doctor is working out what the patient thinks about her blood pressure and how she feels about taking tablets, rather than being more direct with his own views. This is not always effective, since she might not feel able to say what she thinks, but where the patient feels that they can contribute in this way, the consultation can flow well, moving seamlessly from decision into action, with the patient taking the lead and the doctor affirming the plan. By simply confirming that weight can contribute to high blood pressure, and encouraging the patient to compare how she feels about trying to lose weight with taking an additional tablet, the doctor has helped to enable a commitment to behavioural change (notwithstanding that deciding to lose weight and achieving this are far from the same thing!). He may be able to increase her motivation by the reference to her knees – framing her idea of weight loss as something positive for her knees rather than blaming her knee pain on her weight.

Doctor: *"So let's watch things for now and see how you get on. How long do you think we should leave it?"*

Patient: *"I don't know, six months?"*

Doctor: *"I think that would be about right. Perhaps we could review it then, and if it's about the same then we could have another think about tablets?"*

Patient: *"That sounds good."*

Doctor: *"What about your knees, would you like us to do any more about them?"*

Patient: *"Oh, I think it's old age. They're not too bad really."*

Doctor: *"Have you wanted to take a painkiller for them?"*

Patient: *"No, they're never that bad."*

Doctor: *"OK, I think it's fine to watch, but if they are getting too much then the next step might be to get them X-rayed to see how much wear and tear there might be."*

Having come up with a plan for the blood pressure, the doctor returns to the problem of the knees. He has already established that there is no significant medical concern about her knees, so he is looking at optional rooms and wants to test the ground of what she is looking for. By saying *"They're not too bad really,"* the patient is steering away from looking for a solution, but is that because she thinks the only solution is a knee replacement? Would she be interested in something simpler? For this reason the doctor opens the door to the painkiller room and invites the patient to have a look inside, asking *"Have you wanted to take a painkiller for them?"* Since she is happy to move on without exploring this room, the doctor can simply signal where he might think about going if the situation changes, leaving ajar the room marked 'X-ray' to come back to at a later stage if needed.

Medication reviews frequently involve chronic disease management and so lack the basic structure of a newly presenting problem. It can be like picking up a book and starting somewhere in the middle which, again, creates a challenge for a consultation model to follow, particularly if it has a linear structure. The basic tenets of working out what matters and deciding together what to do about it still apply, however, and to bear in mind that most of these consultations take place in the garden can help to keep the patient at the centre of decisions. The garden only rarely encompasses medically urgent or immediately life-threatening situations and so can usually be considered to be a series of optional rooms. The doctor's role is to help the patient weigh the importance of the information being considered – how bad is my blood pressure? What will happen if I do nothing about my early diabetes? How worried should I be about my drinking? – so that options can be considered in an informed way and in keeping with what matters to the patient. There are times when other rooms will need to be explored, however. For instance, Room 101 might be encountered when someone's diabetes has reached the point where insulin should be considered, or an empty room might have to be navigated when someone has pinned their hopes on an effective medication to help them lose weight.

> **Medication reviews can be like picking up a book and starting somewhere in the middle**

Of course, not all medication reviews revolve around chronic disease management or disease prevention. Some of the most challenging in terms of structure are with ongoing mental health problems. A new trainee might be comfortable with an initial presentation of depression, for instance, but unsure what to talk about the second or third time they see the same patient. They may feel they have made all the decisions about medication or talking therapy and have run out of actions to take, and so the consultation can lose all sense of purpose and structure. Asking what it is that matters today can help to bring a sense of order. This may be in the form of a direct question to the patient (for instance, *"What would you like to focus on today?"*) or a question the doctor tries to answer internally as the consultation progresses. Having already visited the patient's *House of Discovery* once or twice in the preceding consultations, what is left to explore? Are there any new changes to the house that need to be considered, such as new symptoms or a change in circumstances? Or are there areas of the house that were not considered last time and would be valuable to look at now? For instance, it may be that the impact of the problem on home life was neglected last time since the focus was on stress at work; or perhaps the patient now trusts the doctor enough to allow a trip to the basement and they are ready to open up about areas of their life that have previously been hard to share.

A consultation model for miscellany

There are undoubtedly odd things that come our way in general practice, and we can dismiss some encounters as not being a 'proper' consultation. One patient may attend just for a sick note or for a medical form to be signed; another makes an appointment because they have noticed bizarre lumps at the back of their throat and are worried that something serious must be wrong, when they have only seen ordinary tonsils; or an angry patient just comes to make a complaint. It is certainly commonplace for a patient not to have a 'presenting problem' to consider, and yet the same principles of the *Two Houses* model can apply and we can ask ourselves the same questions: What matters? Can we achieve a shared understanding? What shall we agree to do about it? Which rooms might I expect to encounter?

For instance, if all a patient needs is to have a form signed then to establish that this is what matters, and (where appropriate) agree to sign it (or where inappropriate, to recognise that we are facing an empty room), may be all that is needed for an entirely successful consultation – one that we might feel could have been done more efficiently than in a face-to-face encounter, of course, but a successful one nevertheless. What is more, since such a consultation may be very brief, it could present a perfect opportunity to get some good gardening done; the patient may well be very grateful for the extra attention of a blood pressure check and some healthy lifestyle advice, for instance.

What about the young person and their healthy tonsils? I think I see this presentation about every other year; sometimes it is their tonsils that have alarmed them, sometimes it is the odd-looking papillae at the back of the tongue; it is not surprising that this crops up from time to time, since the pharynx is an odd-looking thing that we rarely look at. Once we realise that the patient's priority is to understand what they are seeing, we know that we will want to spend most of our time in the *Increased Understanding* wing of the *House of Decision*. There will be technical information to impart, meaning we will want to visit the High Tech Room, and since this will not be the last time that we will need to explain normal pharyngeal anatomy to a patient, it will be worth our while refining a good technique to do this. Initially I found it surprisingly hard to convince patients that what they were seeing was normal until I hit upon the idea of using Google Images of normal tonsils, something that works every time and helps patients to leave the consulting room both reassured and empowered.

With the angry patient we will certainly want to apply the principles of *Popping the bubble* (see *Chapter 5*) and we may also do well to consider whether there is an empty room to negotiate. It may be that their wish is to see a doctor struck off, or a staff member sacked, when such action would be grossly disproportionate, or against employment law. Seeing such a demand as an empty room to be understood and explored with the patient rather than simply resisted may help to defuse the situation, while looking for a hidden room – such as the proactive way the practice would want to learn from such a complaint by conducting a learning event review – may help further.

There are certainly some consultations where nothing appears to have been achieved, and yet it still seems to help the patient. Seemingly insoluble problems were talked about, no decisions were made and no action taken, but the patient still seems to have benefited. Undoubtedly, such encounters can seem very unstructured and are hard to fit to a consultation model, nor should we try to shoehorn a consultation into a particular model just so that we can feel better about it. Even here, however, it may be helpful to consider that the most useful thing the doctor can do is to remain interested and curious in the *House of Discovery*, resisting the urge to rush on to the second house in an effort to fix things. It may be that what really matters is for the patient to have their story heard, and that they wish to tell the doctor of their problems so that they feel understood, but have no desire to visit the *Solutions* wing of the *House of Decision*. An understanding of the power of Narrative Medicine[1] can come to the fore here.

> **Seemingly insoluble problems were talked about, no decisions were made and no action taken, but the patient still seems to have benefited**

When it comes to managing different clinical conditions in the consultation, patterns emerge within the model where the same issues arise again and again, and their place within the rooms of the two houses becomes both more familiar and easier to anticipate. With a good medical understanding of the specific conditions underpinning many of our consultations, working models can be developed to help us approach many of the problems we are faced with, and this will be the subject of the next chapter with the introduction of the *Two Houses Guides* to the consultation.

---

1. Launer, J. (2018) *Narrative-Based Practice in Health and Social Care: conversations inviting change*, 2nd edition. Routledge.

Chapter 16

The *Two Houses* guide to passing the CSA

If you are a GP trainee and have yet to get through the hurdle of the Clinical Skills Assessment (CSA) then you may well have picked up this book, looked at the contents page and headed straight for this chapter. If so, then I can't say I blame you! No matter how much someone wants to learn the art of being a really good GP, they have to actually become a GP in the first place, and the CSA is a daunting obstacle to overcome; it is no wonder that it dominates the mind until it has been passed. A very reasonable critique of any consultation model, therefore, is to ask, "How will it help me pass the CSA?" and the *Two Houses* model needs to be able to answer this question.

I have had debates with trainees over the years about the best way to prepare for the CSA and, as so often happens with trainees, my discussions with them have made me change my mind. We have often talked about how much reading they should do in the form of revision; I used to advise them to do very little; it is a practical examination after all, and the best way to prepare for it is to see patients and gain experience. What coloured my view is how most trainers would feel about sitting the CSA, compared with the Applied Knowledge Test (AKT). Ask most trainers how they would feel about sitting the AKT and we start quivering at the very thought; we know that we would have to spend hours reading the latest knowledge updates to acquire the hard facts needed to sit such a rigorous multiple choice (MCQ) examination. By contrast, if we had to sit the CSA, while we would not relish the idea, most trainers would sit it tomorrow if they had to, and without any preparation. What trainees have impressed upon me over the years, however, is that it is all very well for trainers to say this; it is very different for them. Since a full-time GP conducts roughly 5000 consultations per year, a trainer with 10 years' experience has vastly more experience than a trainee, who may have fewer than 2000 appointments in total under their belt by the time they are expected to sit the CSA. The trainer is unlikely to have anything come up in the examination that they have not dealt with before, while the trainee will inevitably be left with gaps in their knowledge. To encounter a condition for the first time in the CSA is a daunting prospect indeed and so there must be a role for some sort of reading and revision to fill these gaps.

Nevertheless, the fact that trainers feel so differently about the AKT and the CSA is worthy of note, and implies that there should be a different way to approach these two exams, and to acquire the required knowledge base for each. I'm reminded of a time when I debriefed with a trainee of mine after she sat the CSA. She was remembering the cases she had been faced with, recalling which had seemed to go well and which ones she was worried about; one case was easy, she said, because it was just someone presenting with atrial fibrillation (AF). We then remembered that four months earlier, AF had been something of a *bête noire*; she had seen a patient with new-onset AF and been completely flummoxed, not knowing how to start with all the issues she had to cover. We had gone through the case together at the time and then covered AF in a tutorial, looking at the 'jobbing GP' approach to AF rather than referring to guidelines. We covered issues such as when to consider hospital admission, how to balance rate control against rhythm control, how to discuss anticoagulation, what the patient might be thinking or afraid of, when to refer to cardiology, and so on. Soon after this she had seen another patient with AF and this had been sufficient to so embed her own practical approach to AF that she thought it was easy when it came to the CSA, completely forgetting how difficult she used to find it. What was unfamiliar ground had become 'home turf', an area of competence and confidence.

> **What was unfamiliar ground had become 'home turf', an area of competence and confidence**

The approach to the CSA must be similar; an attempt to achieve a practical, working understanding of a topic rather than a detailed knowledge of all the minutiae that might be needed for a written examination. In the AKT the examinee has no control over what might come up, and so needs to know the guidelines in great detail in order to cover all their bases; the facts are presented in the stark, black and white choices of an MCQ, with no room for interpretation or nuance. In the CSA the examinee has much more control; they can steer the consultation towards their areas of strength, and neither the actor nor the examiner is going to be concerned with minutiae; it is about broad strokes, covering them well and working with the patient rather than detailed knowledge of guidelines. It does still depend on secure foundational knowledge, however, and, despite my previous protestations to the opposite, the trainee will still need to do some background reading and preparation.

There is no substitute for seeing patients, and this remains the cornerstone of CSA preparation, but it needs to be backed up by appropriate reading and planning, especially when real-life patients have been seen and this reveals a gap in understanding – as with my trainee and her first case of AF – or when a trainee has simply not seen many patients with a particular problem.

The trainee needs to build up a mental, practical portfolio of working models for different scenarios that might be encountered in the consultation, whether it is a specific clinical condition such as AF, a broader theme such as an issue relating to genetic testing, or a scenario such as dealing with an angry patient or a concerned relative. The *Two Houses*

> **The trainee needs to build up a mental, practical portfolio of working models for different scenarios**

model can give a practical framework for building up this portfolio and I have developed *Two Houses Guides* to help with this, as a free resource for trainees who would like to use the model for this purpose.

Each *Two Houses Guide* considers a specific scenario that might come up in the examination (or, of course, in real life) and asks the questions that we might want to consider when encountering this problem. Questions such as:

- What is likely to matter to the patient?
- What should matter to the doctor when faced with this scenario?
- Are there particular rooms we might need to explore in the *House of Discovery*? Do we need to consider what might lie in *the Basement*? Might we expect to find *Dry Rot*? Is there anything we should tend in *the Garden*?
- Are there rooms to look out for in the *House of Decision?* Are there *Empty Rooms* or *Locked Rooms* that might trip us up? Might there be a *Hidden Room* we could utilise? Is there going to be a *Room 101?* What are the main *Optional Rooms* that will be available for this problem?
- How should we navigate the *High Tech Room?*
- What will we need to consider when *Forecasting* what might happen next?
- What might we put in our *Toolbox* to help us with this scenario?
- Underpinning all of this, what are the broad strokes of *Foundational Knowledge* that our consultation will depend upon?

The *Two Houses Guide to the Menopause* is available online at www.scionpublishing.com/TwoHouses in an A4 format that can easily be printed off; a smaller version is shown below.

Two Houses Guide Example 1

The menopause is a good example of a scenario where the trainee may well have gaps in their knowledge; it is rarely encountered in a hospital setting, even in gynaecology clinics, and many trainees will approach their CSA without ever having started someone on hormone replacement therapy.

A *Two Houses* consultation guide

Managing the menopause

The House of Discovery: work out what matters

To the patient

How does she feel about being menopausal? Is fertility an issue?

Does she want confirmation of the menopause, general advice, or is she looking for treatment of symptoms?

Which symptoms bother her the most? This will guide which treatment you might consider – HRT is best for flushing, topical oestrogen for dryness, maybe antidepressants or CBT if primarily a mood problem.

What are her views on HRT? Are there any personal, friend or family stories that have influenced her?

Simply asking 'what do you think about HRT?' can be a great way to start this conversation. What does she think about alternative treatments? You might not want to initiate the idea of alternatives, but it is helpful to explore if it is on her agenda.

To the doctor

Is it the menopause, or something else? Heavy or frequent periods may be due to the menopause, but there are many other causes.

Red flag symptoms? (see below)

Does she need contraception? (see below)

Are there contraindications / cautions to HRT? There are few absolute CI to HRT (breast cancer being the main one), but it is important to consider risk of breast cancer, risk of VTE and CVD. Might need bloods to assess CVD or VTE risk if there is a strong family history or personal risk factors.

Need to check her blood pressure before starting HRT.

What to look out for in the *House of Discovery*

Finding Dry Rot

There are two main areas where you might uncover unexpected bad news, so you need to be ready for them.

You suspect the menopause, but she has not considered it. If this is premature then this could clearly be bad news, esp. if family not complete, but even if normal age it can be an unwelcome milestone of ageing.

She has assumed it is the menopause, but symptoms are more worrying and a Two Week Rule referral is needed.

Tools for the toolbox

"How would you feel if this was the menopause?"

"Did you just want to know if this was the menopause, or did you want to talk about how we might treat your symptoms?"

"What do you think about HRT?"

"Which symptoms bother you the most?"

Tending the Garden

You need to consider CVD risk when prescribing HRT, so this is a good time to see if this needs attention.

Is her BP OK?

Does she smoke?

Is weight an issue?

If you are doing blood tests, would it be an opportune time to check lipids/HbA1c?

Foundations

Based on 2017 NICE CKS on the menopause and MHRA Update August 2019 following key study in *The Lancet*.

Key symptoms of the peri-menopause: Change to menstrual cycle (usually fewer periods, but could be more frequent), flushing, night sweats, joint pains, mood and sleep disturbance, including an increase in restless legs syndrome, sexual dysfunction.

Key symptoms of post-menopausal state: Absence of periods, vaginal dryness, weakness of pelvic floor.

Investigations: These are **not** usually needed as the menopause is a clinical diagnosis. Consider FSH/LH/oestradiol in women <45 when symptoms are atypical, or if using a Mirena coil as amenorrhea occurs anyway. Impossible to interpret when taking oestrogens (e.g. when on HRT or combined pill) and guidance unclear about value when on progesterone alone.

Symptoms to investigate: If age >45, a sudden change in bleeding pattern, irregular or post-coital bleeding usually needs referral (Two Week Rule if cervix looks abnormal). Post-menopausal bleeding needs Two Week Rule Referral.

Contraception: A woman can be considered infertile due to the menopause once she is 55 years old, or has had 2 years without a period if <50 years, or 1 year without a period if aged >50 years. HRT does **not** provide contraception.

Disclaimer: Two Houses Guides are intended to give a practical basis to structure a consultation and are not a substitute for consulting the latest clinical guideline.

A *Two Houses* consultation guide

Managing the menopause

The House of Decision: decide together what to do

Rooms to look out for

Empty Rooms

Patients can expect too much from 'hormone' blood tests, when testing FSH/LH is purely binary – it tells you if you are at the menopause or not, but nothing more.

Hidden Rooms

Alternative treatments for menopausal flushing – e.g. black cohosh. Some women will have heard of these, some will be unaware – what do you think of it as a doctor? Those that work probably contain phytoestrogens.

Room 101

How does she feel about HRT? If this is premature menopause (age <40) then declining HRT could have significant implications for bone strength. If she is worried about HRT it might help her to see that you would only be taking her up to the natural age of the menopause, and breast cancer risk only really starts by extending the exposure to hormones well beyond 50. Help her to balance the risks of HRT with the risk of osteoporosis – does she have family members affected by this?

Key decisions in the *House of Decision*

Are investigations needed?

See *Foundations* for straightforward menopause, but are there any odd symptoms that don't fit and might need looking into?

HRT or not? Which type of HRT?

HRT is for quality of life reasons and only has prognostic benefits in premature menopause. Don't forget lifestyle changes/CBT/SSRIs. See *Foundations* for whether to use oral or patches. Route of administration (oral / transdermal) has no bearing on breast cancer risk.

Contraception needed?

If so then the Mirena coil and systemic oestrogen can be ideal, but the idea of a coil is a very personal one. Remember that the combined pill will work as both contraception and HRT, so is a great alternative to HRT in younger women who need contraception and are low risk.

How long to use HRT for?

Generally 3–5 years, but depends on QOL when coming off it. No upper age limit if prepared to take the risks, especially with oestrogen only.

The High Tech Room

Difference between peri- and post-menopause

You could describe the first as the ovaries misbehaving and sending out hormones in a random way, and the latter as the ovaries going to sleep.

Purpose of treatment

Important to know that it is fine to go through a natural menopause, but also that treatment can really improve quality of life – which is the only reason to consider HRT.

There is a lot to explain in respect to the menopause – don't overload her! Here are key messages to get across:

Explaining risks of HRT

How to share this – you could use Cates plots, or could just have some of the key numbers to hand. Some women will want actual numbers, others will prefer to know if risks are big or small. Remember, the risks are due to extending the natural age of the menopause, so HRT under 50 is different to taking it beyond 50.

Risks of HRT

Per 1000 women age 50 for 5 years:

Breast cancer risk is biggest concern

Baseline: 13 cases

Oestrogen-only HRT: +3 cases

Combined sequential HRT: +7 cases

Combined continuous HRT: +10 cases

With 10 years of HRT, risk doubles

Risk of venous thromboembolism

Baseline: 5 cases

Oestrogen-only HRT: +2 cases

Combined HRT: + 7 cases

Other risks very low +1 case of stroke; no increased cardiac risk.

Foundations

Based on 2017 NICE CKS on the menopause and MHRA Update August 2019 following key study in *The Lancet.*

Combined HRT or not: Use unopposed oestrogen if a woman has had a hysterectomy, but otherwise she must have progesterone (either systemic or in a hormonal coil) to prevent irregular bleeding and uterine cancer.

Sequential or continuous HRT: Sequential (with either monthly or 3-monthly bleeds) is best in peri-menopause or she is likely to get abnormal bleeding. Use continuous in post-menopause – but some room for patient preference here when periods are infrequent. Sequential HRT has a slightly lower risk of breast cancer than continuous HRT.

Patches, transdermal gel, oral or vaginal: This is largely patient preference, but patches can be better in some circumstances, e.g. if on enzyme-inducing drugs like carbamazepine. Vaginal oestrogen alone is best for vaginal dryness, and no need to oppose with progesterone. There is no extra risk of breast cancer with topical HRT.

For a model such as this guide to the menopause to really help a trainee it must become a *working* model; the theory needs to be put into practice either in the consulting room, or by practising the scenario in CSA role play. The guide will be most useful, therefore, if the trainee then seeks out a scenario on the menopause to role play and sees how it works in reality. The guide can then become personalised, annotated either mentally in the working model forming in the trainee's memory, or literally by red pen or highlighter on the written guide. If the scenario doesn't work that well first time, find another and try again until the menopause moves from an area of concern to an area of confidence – just like AF did for my trainee earlier in this chapter.

Trainees should avoid the urge to either read endless guidelines devoid of real-life application, or engage in excessive role play without considering any theoretical framework

This combination of reinforcing theory with a practical model, and active practice in the real world or in role play, seems to me to be the best way to prepare for the CSA; avoiding the urge to either read endless guidelines devoid of real-life application, or engage in excessive role play practice without considering any theoretical framework.

The *Two Houses Guide to the Angry Patient* is available online at www.scionpublishing.com/TwoHouses in an A4 format that can easily be printed off; a smaller version is shown below.

Two Houses Guide Example 2

There are some scenarios that will be encountered in the CSA where there are no obvious guidelines to refer to, such as encountering an angry patient, a concerned relative or a general approach to something like a request for genetic testing or alternative therapies. Not that these areas are completely devoid of guidance; the General Medical Council and medical defence unions give some guidance for dealing with complaints, for instance, but, as with much of general practice, there is no neat and tidy guideline to help us. This confirms the value of making our own working models for these problems, and the second example concerns a favourite for the CSA, working with an angry patient.

Two Houses Guides online

The two examples given here are available to download and print at www.scionpublishing.com/TwoHouses. Further *Two Houses Guides*, covering other conditions and scenarios, are available at my website, www.twohousesgp.com. The guides are a free resource to access, download and share, although they are subject to copyright and so should not be shared in an altered form, shared without attribution, or published in another format. Over time more guides will be added, and updates to existing guides will be made where appropriate.

There clearly needs to be a disclaimer for these guides. The foundational knowledge has been based on recent guidelines or considered best practice, but clearly this remains my own interpretation of the latest guidance and is not meant to replace nationally accepted standards. Since best practice is constantly evolving, each guide is only as accurate as it can be at the time it is devised.

Developing your own guides

While I hope the guides I have developed will be helpful, both for the CSA and for understanding how the *Two Houses* model works in real life, for anyone training in primary care who would like to use the *Two Houses* model, there would be great value in developing your own sketched-out guides. These might be for problems you encounter in the consulting room, or for CSA preparation, but by going through the questions listed earlier in this chapter you should be able to develop your own bespoke working model for how you want to approach some of the different clinical scenarios that we are faced with in primary care. As well as helping with the specific setting for which you design the guide, taking the time to develop even a few such guides will help to embed the concepts within the *Two Houses* model. Over time it will become second nature to predict the rooms we might encounter and instinctive to use the consultation skills we need to navigate our way from first meeting the patient on the doorstep of the *House of Discovery*, through the two wings of the *House of Decision*, and all the way to Forecasting the future as we bid them farewell at the Porch.

**A *Two Houses*
consultation guide**

**The angry
patient**

The House of Discovery:
work out what matters

To the patient

What is it that has made them angry? Are they angry with:
- something that has happened?
- the way they have been treated?
- an individual?
- a system or organisation?

Do they want to make a formal complaint, or do they just want to be heard today?

Do they want any direct action other than dealing with the complaint? For instance, new clinical actions to rectify what has happened.

If they are making a complaint, what outcome would they like to result from it? Possibilities include:
- being heard
- an apology
- knowing that steps will be taken to make sure it doesn't happen again
- an investigation into what happened
- a staff member to be disciplined (including being sacked or struck off)
- compensation, be it financial or otherwise.

To be heard, receive an apology and to know learning has occurred are by far the most commonly desired outcomes

To the doctor

Listen, listen, listen. Since the most important thing when you are angry is to feel you have been heard, what must matter most to the doctor is to make sure the patient feels that the doctor has listened. Apologise early and sincerely and agree with the patient whenever you can.

How can the doctor learn from what has happened?

How can the organisation learn?

Respect confidentiality at all times – especially important if someone is complaining on behalf of someone else.

Does the complaint raise issues of probity?

Should an investigation be undertaken?

Would the patient like this to be handled informally, or formally through the complaints system?

Are there unresolved clinical areas that should be addressed in the light of what has happened?

Are there underlying reasons why the patient got so angry? Tread carefully in finding this out, but it may be possible to explore this at an appropriate time.

What to look out for in the *House of Discovery*

Check at every stage

While we would not normally ask for permission to ask simple questions, when the patient is angry it is best to check regularly before proceeding – much as we might before entering the basement.

The Basement

There may be underlying issues for the patient to explore, such as stress at home or anger issues, but resolve the anger first before going there!

Tools for the toolbox

"I'm really sorry this has happened."

"I'm very sorry to hear that; can you tell me a bit more about what went wrong?"

"You are quite right, this shouldn't have happened. We will want to see what we can learn from this."

"What can I do to help here?"

Popping the bubble

The priority when faced with an angry patient is to bring down the level of emotion, so that doctor and patient can then communicate more effectively. An early and sincere apology can really help to 'pop' the angry bubble. Keep your own voice calm and your body language open; make it clear that you are concerned about what has happened and you will do your best to try to improve the situation; avoid being defensive.

Foundations

Based on British Medical Association advice on handling complaints in primary care.

Practice complaints policy: Every practice must have a complaints policy and a named responsible person (usually a partner or the practice manager) who is responsible for

handling complaints. All formal complaints should go through this person, or a deputy if they are away. Be familiar with your own practice policy.

Making a complaint: While patients should be asked if they would like to make the complaint in writing, they **do not have to do so**. The practice is obliged to respond to the complaint as part of

its contractual responsibility and most complaints are dealt with in-house without reference to an outside organisation.

Timescales: Practices must acknowledge a complaint, either verbally or in writing, within 3 days. After this there is no strict timetable, but it should be dealt with as quickly as possible and the patient kept informed if there are any delays.

Disclaimer: Two Houses Guides are intended to give a practical basis to structure a consultation and are not a substitute for consulting the latest clinical guideline.

**A *Two Houses*
consultation guide**

**The angry
patient**

The House of Decision:
decide together what to do

Rooms to look out for

Empty Rooms

Sometimes the patient wants an action that is not possible, for instance for the practice to sack a staff member without regard to employment law, or for a doctor to be struck off for a simple mistake. It is important to acknowledge this and understand why they have reason to want this, before explaining why issues such as employment law might prevent such actions being taken.

The patient may expect the complaint to be dealt with in an unrealistic timescale; for instance, if a key staff member involved in the complaint is on holiday, any investigation may have to wait until they return.

Hidden Rooms

Most patients would like to know that the organisation will learn from mistakes so that they won't be repeated. Many may be unaware, however, of systems such as Learning Event Analysis, Serious Untoward Incident reviews, or national reporting schemes (NRLS, see *Foundations*). For the doctor to offer these as unexpected ways that the organisation might use to try to learn can often show listening in action and not just in words.

There are other organisations that can help, especially if the complaint is against another part of the NHS (see *Foundations*)

Key decisions in the *House of Decision*

Would the patient like this to be dealt with as a formal complaint? If so, would they like to complain verbally, or to put it in writing? A complaint is often dealt with more completely if submitted in writing, but **do not insist on this** (see *Foundations*).

Would it help to explain the complaints system?

If you need to speak to someone else in the practice, do you have the patient's permission to do so?

How would the patient like the practice to respond to the complaint? There will probably need to be an investigation, so would they like to hear the results of this, and if so, would they like to receive a letter, or to arrange a meeting?

Does there need to be any involvement of another organisation, such as the hospital, or social services? If so, should the practice help, or is there another body that would be better placed to help here? (see *Foundations*).

Ensuring closure

Gaining understanding

As well as wanting to be heard, the patient may want to leave with a greater understanding of what went wrong. The challenge is for the doctor to explain errors or problems without getting defensive.

It is also important to be honest about where colleagues might have gone wrong, without overtly blaming someone who is not there to defend themselves, or seeming to close ranks as a profession against the patient.

Tools for the toolbox

"We take complaints very seriously and I am very happy to put this through our formal complaints process, would that be helpful?"

"How does that sound to you?"

"So, to summarise, I am going to look into what has happened here with the help of our practice manager and Dr Ahmed who is our complaints lead; we will write to you within 2 weeks."

Forecasting

Check carefully that the patient is happy with the outcome you have agreed to and the timescale by which the next step will be completed.

Make sure that the patient knows how to approach the practice again if they are unhappy with the way any complaint is being handled, and that they know they can take the complaint to the Ombudsman if they are unhappy with the outcome (see *Foundations*).

Foundations

based on 'How to Complain to the NHS' Government website.

Other organisations that can help patients with a complaint: Patient Advice and Liaison Service (PALS – every NHS Trust has one): For problems with hospital care, lost appointments, etc., especially if urgent clinical need.

NHS Advocacy Service: Can provide advice and advocacy support in making a complaint against any part of the NHS.

NHS England and the GMC: Patients can complain directly to either of these organisations, but both usually pass the complaint back to the practice in the first instance. If they are unhappy with the outcome of the complaint then they can

appeal to the Parliamentary and Health Service Ombudsman, and practices are obliged to make this known to them.

National Reporting and Learning System (NRLS): This is a system where doctors can report when things went wrong, so that learning can be shared nationally and mistakes can be reduced in future.

Disclaimer: *Two Houses Guides* are intended to give a practical basis to structure a consultation and are not a substitute for consulting the latest clinical guideline.

Chapter 17

Consulting in the 21st century

Much has changed since Pendleton and Neighbour wrote their seminal works on the consultation. The make-up of the primary care team has altered profoundly, the telephone is used more than ever as the first point of contact, and digital consulting has become a reality. Any attempt to reimagine the consultation must, therefore, take account of these developments and seek to both embrace and inform the future shape of general practice. In the final chapter of this book I would like to ask what a broader, multi-professional team means for the consultation, and to consider the opportunities, challenges and threats of both the telephone and the digital revolution on the consultation.

The COVID-19 pandemic hit the UK after the first proofs of this book had been completed and thrust change upon general practice and the whole of world society with its arrival. There is no doubt that it has turned the whole of general practice upside down in the short term, demonstrating just how adaptable primary care can be in a crisis. In the space of a few days most practices went from a majority of face-to-face appointments to consulting almost entirely by telephone or video, an overnight transformation the like of which none of us has ever known. What the face of general practice will look like when this has all settled down is totally unknown at the time I am writing this addition to the proofs.

They say that necessity is the mother of invention, and there has certainly been a seismic shift in the use of technology to enable remote consulting; prior to the start of March 2020, practices that were able to offer video consulting, for instance, were in a small minority; by the end of the month almost every practice had this capacity and most GPs had tried it out, usually with good results. Digital platforms are being rolled out at speed, and it remains to be seen if this is just the impetus the profession needed to modernise, or if we will have to backtrack because poorly thought-out systems have been put into practice.

There has already been a great deal of human and social cost in terms of lives lost and businesses collapsing, with the prospect of ripples of grief, fear and the effects of poverty that will inevitably follow in the wake of the virus. One thing we can be sure of is that general practice will be there when this is over, ready to sit in the rubble with our patients as we try to help them rebuild their lives. There will be positive developments for the profession from this most challenging of times, but there will also be those who will use this experience to argue that face-to-face consulting is old-fashioned and inefficient, and this must be resisted robustly if we are to defend the values of our profession. Technological advances are greatly to be welcomed, as long as they remain wedded to the values of patient-centred medicine, and enhance rather than detract from what it means to be human.

The multi-professional team

Throughout this book I have referred consistently to doctors and GPs, while being constantly mindful that the scope of practitioners engaging in primary care consulting today is no longer limited to doctors. I considered changing the language I used; perhaps the role of the practitioner could vary throughout the text, or I could always refer to 'practitioners' in a generic sense, but both ideas seemed clumsy. In the end I opted for consistency and for the world I know best – that of GP training. Despite this, it is my very great hope that this book will be read by other healthcare professionals in primary care, since the model I have described (and I think this applies to any consultation model in primary care) is not a *medical* model, but a *primary care* model.

> **What defines a typical GP appointment is not the presence of a doctor as opposed to another healthcare practitioner, but its unscripted nature**

When a nurse sees a patient for a traditional nursing appointment, such as a dressing for instance, or a paramedic responds to a 999 call, they are either seeing a patient with a predefined and specific problem, or a different cohort of patients to the typical GP appointment. It makes sense, therefore, that the consultation model for such appointments may be different to the model a GP uses, although there will always be a great deal of overlap. What defines a typical GP appointment is not the presence of a doctor as opposed to another healthcare practitioner, but the unscripted nature of what the patient brings to the consultation. One of the delights of general practice is that the next patient could be one day old, or one hundred years old; they might bring something as trivial as a verruca or as serious as sepsis; they may be frustrated with unresolving symptoms, or burst into tears the moment they sit down because their life seems to be falling apart. Anything and everything can come through the door.

I well remember in my own GP training the revelatory moment when I realised that, for the first time as a doctor, I genuinely needed to ask the patient, *"How can I help?"* During my six years working in secondary care I had never needed to ask that question. I always knew why the patient was there, because another doctor – either a GP or a doctor in Accident and Emergency – had asked me to see them about a particular problem. It is the unfiltered nature of what we see in primary care that defines it, and so shapes the consultation skills that we need to develop. If consultation models are any help at all in developing these skills, then they should be relevant to all practitioners who engage in the frontline nature of consulting in primary care.

The widening of the primary care healthcare team is to be greatly welcomed, and the very survival of general practice may well depend on it, but it does raise important questions for training within primary care. The main emphasis of the medical curriculum remains the accumulation of medical knowledge rather than the teaching of communication skills, and so there is no reason to think that doctors have any form of head start when it comes to being good communicators. One of the great strengths of general practice, however, is the long-established apprenticeship model for GP training. The luxury of regular one-to-one tutorials, half-day release schemes and formative feedback through directly observed or video consultations provides a fertile environment for the development of good communication skills. The challenge for those responsible for training nurses, paramedics and physician associates in primary care is to show commitment to the teaching of communication skills in a similar way. If we conclude that consultation models are just as important for all practitioners on the front line in primary care, then who is teaching these models to non-GPs? Since I am only involved in the training of GPs, I am unable to answer how well this is taught, or whose responsibility it is to ensure it is done well, but it is important that anyone asked to engage in the challenging task of communicating in primary care is properly equipped with the skills they need to thrive in such an environment.

Telephone triage

There is nothing new about using the telephone in primary care, although the fact that most of us have a phone with us at all times these days has certainly made it increasingly important as a convenient means of communication for both doctor and patient. What has become much more commonplace over the last decade is the use of telephone triage, where the doctor makes an initial assessment of the problem over the telephone.

The nature of this triage 'consultation' is worth examining, since it has similarities to a traditional face-to-face consultation but with one fundamental difference, which is the nature of triage. With triage the objective remains to work out what matters, but the first question is what matters *in terms of triage* rather than anything more detailed. All the doctor and patient need to work out is whether this is something that can be dealt with entirely on the telephone, or whether a face-to-face appointment would be preferable, and then to make a decision about the timing of that appointment and the best person for the patient to see. This can lead to appropriately brief encounters. For instance, if it is clear that a child has an acute illness and it will be important to examine them, but they are quite well enough to wait for the appointment that is available in a couple of hours' time, then the consultation can end in less than a minute with the very satisfactory outcome of an appointment with another healthcare professional who will explore the problem more fully.

Trainees can find such brevity challenging, since it seems incomplete and as though they have not taken a 'proper history'; it feels like a poor handover for which they would be roundly chastised in a hospital setting, or as though they are passing the problem on to someone else without bothering to do an assessment themselves. However, it is important that such triage is kept brief, partly for the sake of efficiency – as there will be many more calls to make – but also so as not to overly influence the outcome of the ensuing consultation. There is something of the nature of walking on freshly fallen snow when exploring the *House of Discovery* with the patient and if someone else treads all over the snow before you then it will inevitably change the nature of the consultation. The patient will have to go over their problem more than

> **There is something of the nature of walking on freshly fallen snow when exploring the *House of Discovery* with the patient**

once, which will impact the telling of their story, while the approach of the person doing triage may be different to that of the practitioner the patient eventually sees, leading to expectations that cannot be met, or tensions that were unnecessary.

Where the outcome of the initial triage is that the problem can be dealt with on the telephone then the full nature of the consultation ensues, with the need to explore the two houses in much the same way as in a face-to-face consultation. The convenience of such an outcome for both doctor and patient, however, must not cloud the fact that it is difficult to communicate well on the telephone. It is well known that telephone consulting is higher risk than seeing someone in person. The lack of ability to examine the patient is an obvious drawback, but even when examination is not required, the biggest challenge on the telephone is that it is much more difficult for doctor and patient to remain 'in hold', to use the dance analogy explored in *Chapter 3*. The lack of non-verbal communication, the frequency with which both parties may try to speak at once, or times when one party remains silent for a while and the other is not sure if they are listening carefully or the line has disconnected, all conspire against effective communication. The doctor needs to be aware that they are deprived of many of the usual cues that tell them if the patient remains with them, especially when exploring the *House of Decision*, and will need to check in with them more often with questions such as *"How does that sound?"* in order to make sure they are on track. There must be a willingness to change course if there appears to be distance developing between doctor and patient – even reviewing the outcome of the triage and leading to a face-to-face consultation after all.

Video consulting

The idea of video consulting has been promoted with great enthusiasm by at least two health secretaries in recent years; it seems glitzy, high tech and modern and makes the politicians seem forward-thinking compared to doctors stuck in the Dark Ages. The question we should ask, though, is why, before the COVID-19 pandemic, it hadn't taken off. The technology is not that modern and many of us are used to communicating with distant relatives or children living away from home via video, yet there is little demand from patients to be able to communicate this way with their doctor. Although as many as 50% of patients say they would like to be able to access video consulting in theory[1], in practice uptake is far lower; for instance, one popular provider of digital consultations in general practice, *Ask My GP*, has consistently found that <0.1% of patients ask for a video consultation as their preferred form of contact[2]. The problem is that it struggles to compete in terms of effectiveness and convenience when compared with a face-to-face appointment (less convenient but the most effective) or either the telephone or email (both far more convenient than getting the technology right to have a video call). Spontaneously calling someone on the telephone is a social norm, but a spontaneous video call from your doctor has all the potential of disturbing someone in a socially awkward situation; even with a close family member, video calls will usually be agreed via text

A spontaneous video call from your doctor has all the potential of disturbing someone in a socially awkward situation

beforehand – how do we do that in general practice? What is more, many of us dislike seeing ourselves on camera (just see how trainees react when you ask them to start filming consultations!) and the advantages over a telephone call, such as better understanding of non-verbal communication, are not sufficiently valued to overcome the practical and social challenges of video consulting in most circumstances.

For general use, video consulting has all the hallmarks of a snazzy bit of kit for which enthusiasts are trying to find a use, rather than a neat solution to a pre-existing problem. There are some scenarios where it has clear value of course; for instance when there is something like a rash that could be demonstrable on video and would save a trip to the surgery. I have found it very helpful when having end of life discussions in a patient's home and a family member living abroad can take part via video since it really feels like they are in the room, compared with being on speaker phone. Video consulting has certainly had a part to play during the pandemic, but even here the telephone has dominated. It could also solve a problem in rural settings where a face-to-face consultation is desirable, but the physical distance between doctor and patient makes it impractical. For the most part, however, video is unlikely to ever revolutionise primary care.

1. Johnston, S., MacDougall, M. and McKinstry, B. (2016) The use of video consulting in general practice: semi-structured interviews examining acceptability to patients. *Journal of Innovation in Health Informatics*, **23(2):** 493–500.

2. Ask My GP (2019) Latest figures continue to show low demand for GP video consultations. Available at: bit.ly/2uiuyX9 (accessed February 2020)

It is hard to talk about video consulting without at least some reference to the new model of care provided by Babylon GP at Hand[3], which has put video consultations at the heart of the doctor–patient interaction. This new NHS provider has been controversial in that it seeks to cover a far wider catchment area than traditional practices and uses video consulting as its preferred form of contact, presumably to overcome the physical distance between doctor and patient in their model. The high uptake of video consulting in their model, therefore, is inbuilt to the design of their service rather than indicative of patient preference at that time. Undoubtedly many patients are happy with this service and like to consult in this way, but it does seem to have been designed to suit the business model of the provider rather than to be a patient-centred service, and certainly makes it difficult for patients without a smartphone.

Digital consulting

By contrast to the lack of demand for video, the interest in being able to contact your doctor through an app, a website or via email has grown in recent years and is only likely to increase. We are used to accessing all other services in this way and the expectation is that doctors should be no different; it can be extremely convenient for both patients and doctors, and the question is not *if* we should be emailing our patients, but *how* we should be doing it. Above all, we need to ensure digital consulting is safe, effective and conserves the principles of truly patient-centred medicine.

When I was at a presentation by one of the companies that provide digital platforms for GP practices, the presenter demonstrated the patient experience for the audience, showing the questions they needed to go through in order to submit an online request for contact with a GP. *"If they don't have a computer then you could always get one of your reception staff to go through it with them on the phone,"* he said, *"and then you can be left to do what doctors are good at, which is making decisions."* He lost me in that moment. I managed not to shout or scream, but the idea that the GP should just be presented with all the facts and then make a decision is anathema to me. It runs contrary to the fact that it is in gathering this information by listening to the patient that we can make the best joint decisions. It reminded me of a time when Jeremy Hunt, who happened to be our local MP as well as the Secretary of State for Health at the time, responded to our invitation to visit the practice. He had been won over by a model of healthcare he had seen in the USA which he called "rooming the patient" and was keen to share its merits with us. The patient was seen in a single room, but by more than one healthcare professional. They might be seen by a nurse first, who would take the history, make an assessment and then call in a doctor who would quickly make the decisions and move on to the next room; it might be efficient, but it's not general practice as I know it, or ever want to know it.

There are great advantages with a digital approach, however. For starters, it is time-efficient; the patient can make contact at a time of their choosing rather than wait for the 8am scramble to get an appointment. The doctor, meanwhile, can come in early to get going with emails that have come in overnight if they choose to, or even work remotely. Many patients like the fact that when the digital interface asks them to describe their problem they can take their time to get it right and make sure they say everything they want to without fear of being interrupted, or taking up too much of the doctor's time. If the questions are well worded they can be used to gain information that the doctor might not always have time to ask. For instance, I have already described how doctors may be tempted to give up asking the patient about their expectations, since too often they get an

A strange case of an ear infection

Back in the days before we did telephone triage, patients with an urgent problem would be added to the evening duty surgery. The receptionist would ask if they could tell the doctor what the problem was when they booked the appointment.

I remember calling in a young woman one evening; the receptionist had written 'ear infection' as the reason for the appointment and so I had my auroscope to hand as I called her in. She started with her opening gambit before she sat down.

"I just need some more of my pill," she said. *"I'm going to run out before the weekend and I don't want to get caught out."*

"Sure," I said, trying not to sound too surprised. *"We can certainly sort that out. I think you also mentioned something about an ear problem?"*

"Oh that," she said. *"That was just a lie so that I could get an appointment."*

It took me a moment to get my head around this, but in the end all I could do was laugh and admire her ingenuity. It made me wonder what was so broken about our appointment system that she had felt the need to lie in order to get what she needed.

uninformative answer; if the digital software asks this question then even if the return rate is low, the doctor has not had to invest time in finding this out and so will be gaining information they might have otherwise missed.

What, then, might be the risks to the consultation in taking a digital approach?

People play games

One of the biggest mistakes we can make when interacting with real humans is to expect them to behave like robots. If a robot had symptoms then it would describe them in exactly the same way, time and again, consistently giving the same response to the same questions; ask a human and anything can happen. How we answer will depend on how we are feeling at that moment, how much time we have got, or how many times our computer has crashed before we finally manage to submit the wretched form. If we get the wrong outcome we may play games until we get what we want; we might not lie as brazenly as my patient without an ear infection, but we may well change our story to suit our needs. For instance, if we don't like the computer's advice to call 999 when we answer 'yes' to a question about chest pain, then we might try again with a different answer and see if we get the outcome we were hoping for. Or if we have to go through the process of answering twenty questions every time we want to get in touch with the doctor, we may well decide we have had enough and take ourselves off to Accident and Emergency instead.

> **One of the biggest mistakes we can make when interacting with real humans is to expect them to behave like robots**

There has been a lot of concern about the use of artificial intelligence (AI) in the development of computer algorithms to assess patients. Mostly these systems involve an app asking the patient a series of closed questions about their symptoms, with each answer leading to a subsequent question until the computer yields a response and suggests an outcome. These outcomes can vary from self-help advice to instructions to see a healthcare professional within a certain time frame, or advice to call 999. Most of the concerns have been about safety, with many examples being shared on Twitter of potentially life-threatening scenarios being dismissed as minor illness by the supposedly intelligent computer. These concerns are valid and need to be addressed, as do the opposite concerns that an overly cautious approach can lead to someone with a minor illness being instructed to 'see a GP within two hours', so putting undue pressure on an already stressed system.

Even if the algorithms can be improved, however, there remains a fundamental problem with this AI approach to healthcare: it relies on the use of closed questions, thereby squeezing out any ability for the patient to say what really matters to them. What is more, it assumes that the outcome is the same for every person, thereby ignoring the fundamental difference between illness and disease. Two patients with the same disease will have a very different illness depending on their context. Tennis elbow is a very different illness for a self-employed plasterer, for instance, than for someone who works at a desk; earache matters far more to the person who is due to fly the following day than someone who will be at home all week; a sore throat is a much bigger deal to an opera singer than a librarian.

Digital platforms are at their best when they increase the opportunity for the patient to express themselves and at their worst when they close down the patient's input. Open questions such as, *"What matters to you the most about this problem?"* or *"Is there anything you were particularly concerned about with this problem?"* can be really informative and give the doctor a useful heads-up about what to explore. A few directed closed questions may add value to the report the doctor receives, but the doctor must see the report as just the starter for the conversation. There is no substitute for exploring the *House of Discovery* directly with the patient and if these digital reports tempt us to jump straight into the *House of Decision* we may well do this at our peril, leaving the patient trailing in our wake.

> **Digital platforms are at their best when they increase the opportunity for the patient to express themselves**

Guarding the main thing

Stephen Covey, the author of *The 7 Habits of Highly Effective People*[4] famously encouraged his readers to recognise that, *"the main thing is to keep the main thing the main thing"*. As we consider the future of general practice we must remember that neither the make-up of the primary healthcare team, nor the use of video; neither triage systems nor digital platforms are the main thing. The main thing is that we continue to deliver compassionate, effective healthcare with the patient at the centre of everything we do.

4. Covey, S. (2013) *The 7 Habits of Highly Effective People*. Simon & Schuster UK.

Embracing change in how we do this may well help us to be more effective, and to cope with the huge pressures general practice is under, but we must not let these changes rob of us the essence of primary care.

In closing, I will leave the final words to Roger Neighbour, who, thirty years on, is still championing the core values of general practice. Let's hope we never stop listening to him:

> *"Consulting skills are not a set of circus tricks, like spinning plates or lion taming. They are the expression, in words and behaviour, of our professional values. The consultation is a shop window where we display what we think is important about doctoring. To the patient, it is the litmus test of whether or not we in fact care as much as we say we do."*[5]

5. Neighbour, R. (2019) Yesterday's man? *British Journal of General Practice*, **69(686):** 456–457.